Confessions of an Rx Drug Pusher

Confessions of an Rx Drug Pusher

✦

God's Call to Loving Arms

Gwen Olsen

iUniverse, Inc.
New York Lincoln Shanghai

Confessions of an Rx Drug Pusher
God's Call to Loving Arms

iUniverse books may be ordered through booksellers or by contacting:

iUniverse
2021 Pine Lake Road, Suite 100
Lincoln, NE 68512
www.iuniverse.com
1-800-Authors (1-800-288-4677)

ISBN-13: 978-0-595-35763-5 (pbk)
ISBN-13: 978-0-595-80237-1 (ebk)
ISBN-10: 0-595-35763-6 (pbk)
ISBN-10: 0-595-80237-0 (ebk)

Printed in the United States of America

This book is dedicated in loving memory to my niece,
Megan Leslie Blanchard
Born June 14, 1984
Entered eternal life December 2, 2004

Memorial Web site: www.cookwalden.mem.com

Contents

Acknowledgments

To all of the earth angels who were sent to assist and encourage me with this project, Phuc and David Armstrong, Laurie Carty, Sally Cassell, Jerry Chandler, Kim Coers, Pamela Gandin, Diane Holley, Rob Raucci, and Rev. Ron Scott, I am humbly grateful. You are kindred spirits, and your inspiration meant the world to me.

To my editor, Shea Spindler, who put the spit and polish on my work, and to the iUniverse editorial staff…thank you, thank you, thank you!

To Mom and Dad whose immeasurable love and support has given me the strength of character to speak my truth.

Lastly, to my husband, Rod, who lovingly supported the process and our family while I spent endless weeks and months married to the computer. After twenty years, you are still my best friend!

Introduction

The intent of this book is not to diagnose or treat any illness. It is an autobiography and a commentary on the insidious elements of family dysfunction that are passed from generation to generation, including addiction, alcoholism, child abuse, domestic violence, criminal behavior, illegal substance abuse, and mental illness. It is also an exposé from the experiential point of view of a fifteen-year veteran in the pharmaceutical industry and addresses how excessive prescription drug use contributes to the deterioration of our family's health, our children's minds and, therefore, to the very fabric of American society! The intent is to inform, provoke, and inspire others to take responsibility for their own health and mental well-being as well as support their loved ones in doing the same.

In recent years, the health of our nation has declined rapidly. Even though the United States spends more money per capita on health care than any other country, we have poorer health care outcomes than many underdeveloped nations do. A recent World Health Study ranked us fifteenth among twenty-five industrialized nations (Starfield). No place is this truer than in the health care of our mentally ill. Long-term outcomes of mentally ill patients are much better in countries in which the use of psychoactive medications is less frequent (Whitaker 291).

We are a nation of the under-and uninsured as more employers pass the burden of health insurance to individuals that cannot pay the exorbitant premiums every day. Yet, Americans pay an average of seventy percent more for our prescription drugs than our neighboring countries and western European nations because *our* government refuses to impose pricing restrictions on the pharmaceutical industry (Abramson 48). On the other hand, the pharmaceutical industry has been enjoying enormous profits, specifically three to six times greater than those of other Fortune 500 companies. Despite all the public relations hoopla about the tremendous expense of research and development, the truth is that the industry annually fills its corporate coffers with billions of dollars from the sale of inferior new products that add little (if any) therapeutic value over much cheaper, older drugs that are already available. The Food and Drug Administration (FDA) approved seventy-eight drugs in 2002. Only seventeen contained new, active ingredients. The FDA only deemed seven of those to be improvements over older competitors. Furthermore, not one of those seven drugs came from a U.S. manufacturer. The other seventy-one were variations of older products that offered no therapeutic advantages over other similar therapies. (Angell 17).

I never would have thought of myself as a whistle-blower or political activist of any kind. Like many Americans, I turned a blind eye as the government continued empowering the pharmaceutical industry and taking away more and more of my rights and security. We Americans sacrifice our health in order to pursue high-stress jobs and provide for our families. Yet, when we arrive in our retirement years, we are no longer able to enjoy the physical pursuits we experienced in our youth. We must then spend all of our limited resources to maintain or even repair our ailing minds and bodies.

Prescription drug use has become the third-largest killer of Americans, behind heart disease and cancer. More than 180,000 people die annually from the negative effects of legal drugs (Strand 8-9). Obviously, we are in need of radical change to the American medical paradigm!

I have felt tremendous frustration in my attempts to educate others about the perils lurking in every American's medicine cabinet. People are unwilling to listen or are paralyzed by their need to believe in a corrupt system that promises to find future cures for our greatest medical fears while holding us hostage to its financial demands.

It has been said, "The pen is mightier than the sword." It is with this spirit that I have picked up mine in an attempt to help and inform others. I appeal to those gallant knights in white coats who wield their "swords" poised over prescription pads. Please, help stop the madness! To the rest of you, I implore you to wake up and answer God's call to loving arms. The next victim could be someone you know or love.

"*Any vision—or anything—that is true to life, to the imperatives of creation and evolution, will not be unshakable. We must therefore be willing to get shaken up, to submit ourselves to the dark blossomings of chaos, in order to reap the blessings of growth. Much of this is axiomatic: stress often prompts breakthroughs; crises point toward opportunities; chaos is an integral phase of the creative process; and protest abets the cause of democracy.*"

—**Gregg Levoy**, *Callings*

1

A Nightmare before Christmas: Megan's Story

"Even though I walk through the valley of the shadow of death, I will fear no evil, for you are with me..."

—(Psalms 23:4)

I wasn't prepared to return to the scene of Meg's suicide. It was too soon. The enormity of what had happened was only starting to seep in a little at a time. The family assured me the house was presentable. The cleaning crew had been there the previous day to remove any debris or offending evidence caused by the fire. It was necessary to go back and retrieve some of Meg's photos, music, and personal belongings for the memorial service we would have to celebrate her life.

I braced myself on my father's arm as we entered the house. The first thing I noticed was the melted, plastic Venetian blinds next to the front door. Replaying the EMS report in my mind, I envisioned Meg struggling to open the door with her body engulfed in flames. I had to remind myself to breathe. My eyes next caught the exposed wires hanging from the living room ceiling where the fan used to be. She had first attempted to hang herself by fashioning a rope from her shoe-strings and attaching them to the ceiling fan. The fan gave way to her body's weight, and she was unsuccessful. A broken, decorative, ceramic bowl lay on the table below. The carpeting had been removed anywhere there was fire or blood damage, so it was easy to trace Meg's steps as the horrible scene of her last experience on earth unfolded in my mind's eye.

Feeling weak in the knees and nauseous, I could see my mother and sister, Meg's mom, moving about in the next room, Meg's room. Methodically almost robotically, they were fingering Meg's belongings and surveying the damage. A blood-soaked rag and bandanna found at the foot of her bed on a pile of clothes suggested she may have tended to a head wound caused by the ceiling fan. Next to her bedside were copies of *A Course in Miracles* and the Living Bible. Her

1

mother said she had spent a large portion of the night before on her knees as she prayed at the foot of her bed.

More melted blinds drew my attention as we proceeded to the center bedroom. This room belonged to Hayley, Meg's younger sister. In this room, Meg had poured oil from an angel-shaped lantern over herself and ignited it. The intense heat of the fire had obviously risen to the ceiling as it had melted the blinds into clumps of plastic at the very top on each side.

At some point, Meg had a change of heart and desired to live because she ran into the bathroom and tried extinguishing the fire in the bathtub. Apparently, she was unaware this action would only spread the fire. Still struggling to survive, she had the presence of mind to call 9-1-1 and told them she had set herself on fire. The rescuers stated, when they arrived at the scene, she opened the door and fell backwards onto the coffee table. She never spoke a word. It was approximately a thirty-to thirty-five-minute ride to the burn center at Brackenridge Hospital in Austin. She didn't die until they got there. The coroner said she had second-and third-degree burns over ninety-five percent of her body. Only her feet had been spared. The family sent for dental records for the identification process. Seeing her that way was too horrific for any of us to imagine, much less bear witness to.

Megan's Turbulent Childhood

Meg had a volatile relationship with her mother as she grew up, just as we had with ours. Her father refused to acknowledge his paternity before she was even born, which contributed to both Meg's and my sister's abandonment issues. My sister, Michelle, who was pregnant during her last year of high school, fought endless emotional battles and substance abuse as she raised Meg on her own. She repeatedly chose abusive partners. As a result, most of Meg's life was chaotic and unstable. Even worse, Meg was the victim of two different child molesters, resulting from my sister's problems and absentee parenting. Meg was shuffled about from place to place as my sister ran from her past. She always dragged Meg along. Meg never received therapy for her molestation and told me she felt dirty because of it.

Following the first incident of Meg's abuse, my sister and I were estranged for years. Meg was only three years old at the time. After Michelle continued to live with Meg's abuser, I basically wrote my sister off. It broke my heart to lose contact with Meg, but I could not bear to see her in that environment. Moreover, my sister refused to acknowledge the truth about her addictions and her lover until many years later. In fact, in a drunken rage, she had blamed my husband and called *him* a child molester! My towheaded, incessant, little chatterbox of a niece would grow up before I spent much time with her again.

Meg was a remarkably resilient child and truly gifted in many respects. Just as I had been, she was an overachiever in school. She was also a cheerleader and an athlete. She excelled in theatre, art, music, and poetry. She had a beautiful soprano voice and played the viola and guitar. She drew intricately detailed pictures with artistic flair and wrote passionate lyrics to songs she would strum on the guitar and sing herself. She cared about Mother Earth and had compassion for the poor and needy. She worked with the mentally disabled and volunteered at the local food bank.

Meg was beautiful, inside and out. Her broad, dimpled smile could light up a room! She was tall with blonde hair and sparkling, crystal blue eyes. Nevertheless, she felt ugly. According to her, she didn't fit in. Kids were ruthless in their treatment of her. Moving around so much, she never really had any long-term friendships. She found herself a loner most of the time in school. She wanted desperately to be liked, so she courted the approval of other adults in the absence of her parents' attention.

My sister married when Meg was almost nine years old and appeared to finally settle in to a routine domestic life. She quickly had two more little girls, but her marriage was rocky from the start. Following a severe bout of postpartum depression with her third child, my sister's marriage finally disintegrated. Her obstetrician/gynecologist (ob-gyn) first put her on Paxil and then on Prozac. She and Meg began having explosive, physical fights. My sister kicked Meg out. At the time, Meg was fifteen years old.

Michelle would remain on Prozac for more than two years. Once, with her permission while she was visiting, I telephoned her doctor to voice my concern about symptoms she was exhibiting. I relayed information about our family history that included adverse drug reactions, alcoholism, and diabetes. Michelle was consuming massive amounts of water, urinating frequently, and was very moody when she was hungry (common symptoms of diabetes). She was also clearly hypomanic, as she talked incessantly, required little sleep, and stayed up into the wee hours of the morning. She exhibited a considerable tolerance for alcohol, and had been drinking so heavily during her visit that she couldn't even remember her outrageous drunken behavior. Her doctor was not only uncooperative, but he was insulted that I had dared to question his diagnosis and treatment plan. In essence, he told me to mind my own business! Many months later, I witnessed Michelle experience serious manic episodes with withdrawal after discontinuation of Prozac. She also became a full-blown alcoholic. She suffered blackouts when she drank too much, which was frequent. She became severely hypoglycemic and developed narcissistic personality traits in addition to borderline behaviors. All of these are recorded side effects associated with long-term use of Prozac (Tracy 125, 138, 250-251).

Meg came to Texas to live with my family and enrolled as a sophomore in our local high school. We spent the next six months together. During this time, Meg shared the ongoing saga of her family's dysfunction with me. Feeling so lonely and unloved, she lamented the emotional distance my sister placed between herself and her children. She cried endless hours as we hugged and held one another on the couch in consolation. She wanted so desperately to belong.

That summer, my husband was rushed to the emergency room with an incredible blood pressure reading of 210/160. The doctors were amazed he hadn't had a stroke! He began the long, difficult process of recovery, attempting to find the right drug to control his blood pressure with tolerable side effects. His inability to work put stress on the family finances. Our clergy and doctors agreed Meg had to return to Indiana. My husband could not handle the stress of a troubled teenager in the house. Under the circumstances, it was too risky.

It was not that Meg was such a problem herself. She was a typical teenager with typical issues of acne and prom dates. However, having Meg with us meant dealing with my sister's issues. Even with the physical separation of 1,500 miles, there was no reprieve from the drama. We lived it daily via Meg. Meg felt angry, betrayed, and rejected one more time. Her luck would continue to run out.

Michelle decided to move to Texas herself and packed up her other two children, her ex-husband, and all of their problems. She literally moved into my backyard, my very own neighborhood. My husband freaked out!

The usual chaos ensued. My sister's drinking got out of hand. The police called me after picking her up one night on a DUI. I was stunned when she attacked me, both physically and verbally, on the drive home. Like a frightened animal, she became wild. She clawed, screamed, and cursed uncontrollably as she lunged at me from the backseat of the car, which forced me into the dash. Once again, I washed my hands of my sister. I could not handle her abuse. My anxiety and migraines were returning. These were a warning sign. Stress has a very detrimental effect on my health. Even for minute stressors, much less than the kind my sister brought into my life, my body always signals a four-alarm fire response. I feared I might have a meltdown if I didn't protect myself.

Trying to help a manic, psychotic person (especially an intoxicated one) is like trying to help a wounded badger. In spite of your best intentions to help, you will more than likely get eaten up in the process! A family intervention forced my sister to attend rehab. For a while, she seemed to do better. However, she continued to move indecisively between Indiana and Texas, so Meg went to live with my mother in southern Indiana. That meant starting over at yet another unfamiliar high school, which she did. In spite of it all, she graduated with honors and enrolled at Indiana University, my alma mater, to study premed. Her dream was to become a plastic surgeon and help deformed children.

2

My Own Dark Night of the Soul and a Case of Déjà Vu

Don't Be Afraid of the Dark

*At the blackest ebb of midnight—
not a single star in sight—
there's a still and quiet whisper
of ebony delight…*

*It may appear quite frightening
to those without true faith,
but darkness only serves to show
where light can heal our ways.*

*If you listen in the stillness,
you can hear a voice inside.
It's the steward of the lighthouse
sent to help you through the tide.*

*So, don't tremble as you stumble
down life's dark and narrow path.
Pick up your torch and lantern
and forge on to greater tasks!*

*Take heart in your ability
to navigate at night,
and remember that instinctually
you're headed for the light!*

Gwen Olsen (1992)

December 2, 2004, was the day Meg committed suicide. It was also her biological father's birthday. She didn't leave a note. She didn't say good-bye. She didn't get her Christmas gifts, which were still sitting unwrapped on my closet floor. Only two days before that, the last words she said to me were, "I love you, Aunt Gwen." Then we hung up the phone.

So why do I feel so guilty? Because I knew the drugs she had been given were destroying her mentally and I had promised her that I would not allow her to be further chemically abused. However, when it came right down to it, I was unable to keep that promise because none of the decision makers would listen to me until it was too late. That's the problem with becoming overzealous or passionate about a subject. You risk isolating the very audience you seek to educate.

After fifteen years in the pharmaceutical industry as a sales rep, I have more than an average layman's knowledge about drugs and pharmacology. In fact, the first part of my pharmaceutical career was spent as a hospital rep, educating resident physicians in teaching hospitals about psychiatric drugs, among others. However, the majority of my career was spent as a specialty rep, calling on specialists in cardiology, psychiatry, neurology, orthopedics, obstetrics/gynecology, endocrinology, and so forth. These are the scholars among physicians, so the training I received to work with these doctors was exceptional. It also included many preceptorships in several prestigious teaching institutions.

In addition, I had personal experience to back up my book learning. In 1992, following a divorce, my general practitioner encouraged me to try a newly released antidepressant called Zoloft. Prior to that, I was despondent and lethargic, and I had begun losing weight. It seemed like a reasonable suggestion. I was thirty-three years old, and I had never taken antidepressants before. In just a few days, I started having horrendous side effects, including agitation, jitteriness, racing thoughts, and palpitations. I couldn't drive. I couldn't think. I certainly couldn't work and call on doctors. I called my physician. The doctor called me back and assured me these were not side effects associated with Zoloft. He explained that what I was experiencing was known as agitated depression and my condition was worsening before the drug took effect. He suggested we increase the dose. I complied.

My memory doesn't serve me as to what happened next, but I fortunately kept a journal of my chemically induced foray into madness. Apparently, after doubling the dose, I began experiencing psychotic delusions. I also noted involuntary muscle spasms and an inability to sit still, which I identified to be the neurological side effect known as *akathisia*. I had learned about this devastating side effect while selling Haldol (haloperidol) for schizophrenia and senile dementia. At one point, I curled up in a fetal position to hold myself while I shook uncontrollably, searching for relief from the torturous tremor within. Still, my doctor assured me these types of adverse events were not reported with Zoloft. However, at my insistence, he discontinued the Zoloft therapy. No washout period was given.

He prescribed Prozac next. I stopped journaling two days into my use of Prozac because my hands shook too badly to write and my thoughts raced at lightning speed. The suicidal ideation came in intense and unrelenting urges. I found myself driving up and down Highway 2222 (a curvy, potentially treacherous road), looking for a place to drive off that would appear accidental. I didn't want to leave Austin, my three-year-old son, without the benefit of my insurance. I played out every detail with obsessive compulsion. My once-sharp, brilliant mind was losing touch with reality, and I couldn't bear the psychic pain. Nevertheless, I continued believing in the doctors and the magic pill that would fix my brain chemical imbalance. After all, that's what I was assured the antidepressants would do. Balance my brain chemistry, right?

The list of drugs I was exposed to next is embarrassing, even to a former, die-hard believer of the quick fix. Why I allowed myself to be a guinea pig of that nature is beyond me. However, after three doctors and fourteen pharmaceutical interventions, I had enough! A certain survival instinct kicked in, and I knew my very life was slipping away and my brain was being irreparably damaged. I turned my back on conventional medicine and started an alternative path of healing.

In therapy, I would later liken my harrowing experience with biochemical psychiatry to that of being mentally gang-raped—repeatedly and brutally by men I respected and trusted—then left to die, feeling broken and ashamed because they had convinced me it was my fault and that somehow I had asked for it.

The brain becomes distorted in its functioning as it attempts to overcome the effects of psychiatric drugs. Even when the drugs are stopped, it cannot immediately recover its original functions. In some cases, such as my own, the brain may never fully recover (Breggin and Cohen 47).

After several months on disability and a slow, grueling rehabilitation period, my life returned to some semblance of normalcy. I suffered severe memory loss and decreased cognitive function. This made my profession, much less my daily life, extremely stressful. I lived every moment out of my Franklin Planner. I was fearful I would forget something and fall short of my responsibilities. This created terrible anxiety and social dysfunction, not to mention a negative impact on my self-esteem.

I felt compelled to share with others what had happened to me. Most folks expressed sympathy, but they became uncomfortable when I talked about it. I soon learned to drop the subject. Nobody really seemed to comprehend I had experienced a serious adverse drug reaction that left me permanently brain-damaged. Once you receive a psychiatric diagnosis, everything one says or does becomes suspect, even with loved ones and colleagues.

I developed a natural distrust of pharmaceuticals for depressive disorders and discouraged everyone I knew who was taking them. I felt there was an inherent risk that could not be proven yet. I didn't return to the medical literature for answers until nearly twelve years later when I began researching the subject for Meg. My newly formed interest in natural health and alternative healing had been the focus of my recent years' education, training, and research.

It took another eight years of transition, but I eventually left the pharmaceutical industry disillusioned and, honestly, a little ashamed. My once high-profile, lucrative career now felt like a sham, much like the snake oil peddlers of history. My conscience was ill at ease.

Polypharmacy: Prescription for Drug Interactions

My niece, Meg, then eighteen years old and an honor graduate and premed student at Indiana University, had a similar experience in 2003. Following an automobile accident, Meg was given massive quantities of Vicodin (hydrocodone) and other anti-inflammatory drugs for pain. Her performance at school began waning, and she became depressed.

During exams, Meg decided to take a natural stimulant called ephedra to counteract the sedative effects of her pain medication. She did not know ephedra could be a dangerous drug and it could potentiate or interact negatively with the pharmaceuticals already in her system. She did what is frequently referred to in college as pulling an all-nighter. At some point, she slipped into manic delusions.

Her adverse drug reaction landed her in the psychiatric ward of the local hospital where she received a diagnosis of *bipolar* (manic-depressive) *disorder* and a cocktail of chemicals that would lead to her ultimate demise. Once you are branded with a serious psychiatric diagnosis, it is nearly impossible to receive treatment that does not involve chemical restraint.

Before her death, Meg obtained her pharmacy records for me. Judging from the large quantities of hydrocodone and propoxyphene (both central nervous system depressants) she was taking, I feel certain her initial depressive symptoms were more than likely the result of excessive narcotic drug use. However, because of the number of specialists involved, the doctors never related her depression or any of the subsequent withdrawal symptoms to her drug use. So, they prescribed even more drugs.

The diagnostic criteria listed in the Diagnostic and Statistical Manual of Mental Disorders—Fourth Edition (DSM IV) for sedative, hypnotic, or anxiolytic withdrawal (all of which Meg was prescribed long-term following her car accident) reads as follows:

A. Cessation of (or reduction in) sedative, hypnotic, or anxiolytic use that has been heavy and prolonged.
B. Two (or more) of the following, developing within several hours to a few days after Criterion A:

    1.   autonomic hyperactivity (e.g., sweating or pulse rate greater than 100)

    2.   increased hand tremor

    3.   insomnia

    4.   nausea or vomiting

    5.   transient visual, tactile, or auditory hallucinations or illusions

    6.   psychomotor agitation

    7.   anxiety

    8.   grand mal seizures

C. The symptoms in Criterion B cause clinically significant distress of impairment in social, occupational, or other important areas of functioning.
D. The symptoms are not due to a general medical condition and are not better accounted for by another mental disorder (DSM-IV 147).

When Meg described to me what she felt like, at first on the antidepressants and then later on the antipsychotics they gave her, it mirrored what I had gone through in 1992. This time the initial offending drugs were Zoloft, Paxil, and Effexor XR. As Meg began reacting negatively to each antidepressant, she was either immediately switched to another drug, or additional drugs were prescribed to control adverse side effects.

It is important to elaborate a little here in order to understand how the selective serotonin reuptake inhibitor (SSRI) drugs work in the body. Neurotransmitters are the messengers that relay all of the body's biochemical information between nerve cells. Serotonin is a specific neurotransmitter that affects both mood and impulse regulation and plays an important role in sleep quality. Low serotonin levels are associated with many psychiatric problems. The newer antidepressant drugs work primarily by shutting down select pathways of the brain that remove and recycle neurotransmitters, particularly serotonin. This allows more serotonin to circulate longer between neurons.

There is eminent danger in switching immediately from one SSRI to another. One of the differences between the various SSRI antidepressants is the serotonin receptor that each one affects. While one drug may inhibit reuptake of serotonin and metabolism by one receptor, another inhibits reuptake of serotonin and metabolism by yet another receptor. Because of long-term accumulation, blocking of the receptor can continue long after the drug is stopped. That is where the danger lies. If a patient is given one SSRI and that pathway for the reuptake of serotonin is shut down and then receives a second SSRI without the advantage of a drug washout period, the brain shuts down yet another pathway for serotonin metabolism. Multiple blocking of serotonin pathways can lead to agitation, confusion, and other potentially fatal reactions known as serotonin syndrome. In spite of the potential for serious toxicity, this is a common prescribing practice among doctors (Tracy 97-98).

Meg was simultaneously given narcotic analgesics, nonsteroidal anti-inflammatory drugs (NSAIDs), antidepressants, anxiolytics, antibiotics, muscle relaxants, anticonvulsants, and antipsychotic meds. All were prescribed by well-meaning physicians; however, to the trained eye, it is obvious the left hand did not know what the right hand was doing in this case. Even her pharmacist should have questioned the potential interaction between some of these categories of drugs.

Many of the chemicals she was on are processed through the liver's same enzyme known as the cytochrome P450 system, which controls the breakdown of drugs in the body and their likelihood to interact with other drugs in the system When a person takes a variety of drugs that each use a different enzyme system within the liver, then there shouldn't be a problem. But when a person takes two or more drugs requiring the same enzyme system within the liver to metabolize and eliminate them, then the drugs can be potentiated, that is, made more potent, in the bloodstream and can climb to dangerous levels in their usual doses (Strand 111).

It is also common practice for doctors to prescribe covering antidotes such as Xanax (alprazolam), Valium (diazepam), and Inderal (propanolol) with SSRIs in order to minimize severe neurological agitation or akathisia reactions. In other words, these drugs are prescribed prophylactically because the doctor anticipates adverse side effects from the SSRI. However, all of these antidotes are metabolized by the same cytochrome P450 enzyme and can be potentiated by any of the

SSRIs, or vice-versa. SSRI patients have consistently reported serious adverse reactions to benzodiazepines such as Xanax. Not only does this occur when SSRIs are prescribed in conjunction with the benzodiazepines, it sometimes happens long after the discontinuation of the SSRI and benzodiazepines are reintroduced (Tracy 169).

This partial list of drugs Meg was given within a one-year time frame clearly illustrates the problem at hand: Depakote ER, Seroquel, Vicodin, amoxicillin, penicillin, Desyrel (trazodone), Zoloft, Paxil, Lamictal, Flexeril (cyclobenza-prine), Naproxen, Trileptal, Voltaren (diclofenac), Ultram (tramadol), Effexor XR, Phenazopyridine, Tizanidine, Septra DS, ibuprofen (800 mg), Darvocet N-100 (propoxyphene), Abilify, Zyprexa, Xanaflex (Xanax and Flexeril), and Nabu-metone.

Several of the drugs' package inserts (labels) warn of potential drug interac-tions when used in combination. In fact, all of the following drugs are known to use the cytochrome P450 system in the liver: Darvocet, Effexor, hydrocodone, ibuprofen, naproxen, amoxicillin, Septra DS, penicillin, Paxil, Desyrel, Ultram, Voltaren, Xanax, and Zyprexa (Strand 114).

Meg was never given washout periods between prescriptions in order to mini-mize these risks. The addition of more offending chemicals only added insult to injury in a brain and body struggling to overcome toxicity. Without adequate support, Meg was set adrift on an inflatable "raft with a hole in it" in the vast, deadly sea known as the American health care system. It was inevitable she would eventually perish.

Meg continued struggling with mental and emotional issues. She was forced to drop out of school because she was unable to think clearly and function aca-demically. She became despondent. In addition to taking all of these prescribed drugs, she started abusing illicit street drugs. Unable to work or function physi-cally, she floated from one odd job to another in order to support herself. She was referred from one doctor to another and picked up a new diagnosis following another brief psychiatric referral. This time it would be *schizophrenia.*

In his consultation letter to the referring physician, the psychiatrist concluded the following:

Chief complaints and history:

1.   Chronic Pain

2.   History of MVA (motor vehicle accident) 1 ½ years ago

3. Feels depressed

4. Insomnia

5. Anxiety

Examination:

1. Patient reports of hearing voices and music

2. Patient reports of feeling depressed and hopeless

3. Patient's affect (facial expression) is constricted

4. Denies any current suicidal or homicidal ideations

5. Denies any visual hallucinations

6. Insight and judgment is slightly impaired

Impression:

Based on clinical history and exam, patient's symptoms and signs of the above-altered mental status suggest a possibility of dementia/worsening schizophrenia.

Plan:

MRI of the brain to rule out concurrent possibility of new stroke

1. Zyprexa, 5 mg/PO (by mouth) qhs (one at bedtime) to help with hallucinations and insomnia

2. Paxil CR, 25 mg/PO qd (once daily) for depression

3. Follow-up in four weeks is recommended to assess therapy outcome

What therapy? Meg never received any therapy, at least not counseling where she could sit down with an unbiased third-party human being and just express her fears, cry her tears, lick her wounds, and claim her life. Compassion is what Meg really needed, not more drugs!

Now, Meg would risk exposure to long-term treatment on antipsychotic drugs as well. Note, in the psychiatrist's evaluation, he lists three of the criteria indicated in the symptoms of hypnotic drug dependence and withdrawal: insomnia, anxiety, and auditory hallucinations (hearing voices and music). The following side effects are listed under the Adverse Reactions section of the Vicodin package insert labeled Central Nervous System: drowsiness, mental clouding, lethargy, impairment of mental and physical performance, anxiety, fear, dysphoria (depression), psychic dependence and mood changes (PDR 1357). Therefore, the "depression" and "slightly impaired judgment" he noted could have obviously been caused by the chronic use of high-dose hypnotic drugs. Lastly, his evaluation also clearly states, "Patient denies any suicidal or homicidal ideation." That was before she was given more drugs. Her mental condition rapidly accelerated in its downward spiral.

Meg returned to Texas in late July 2004 after exhausting my mother's patience with her as well. Even the most compassionate people have difficulty being a whipping post. It is hard to imagine how aggressive and out-of-character people behave when reacting adversely to psychiatric drugs. It can be even harder to justify their behavior and to forgive and forget. Once, while swept up in a manic psychotic rage, Meg had threatened my mother with physical violence and burning down her house! I guess we all felt like it was my sister's responsibility to care for her daughter.

Meg had no sooner arrived than my sister had her back in for county mental health services where they prescribed more antipsychotic drugs. This time, it was Zyprexa (15 mg) and Abilify (10 mg). Meg went berserk upon reintroduction to medication. She was extremely agitated and paced incessantly. She didn't want to take the drugs and refused to do so.

"I'd rather die than feel crazy like that, Aunt Gwen! I feel like I'm completely disconnected from myself...you know? Like I'm watching myself from a third-person omniscient point of view." she pleaded for understanding.

Yes, I did know what she meant. I was so torn! I knew exactly how she felt. I had walked in her shoes. I distinctly remembered that feeling of hovering above myself, my logical mind observing the frantic thoughts and compulsive behaviors performed by my disconnected body. The observer self knew everything that was going on, but it could not feel or control anything. I felt powerless over the protagonist. Just like watching a movie, it was surreal. Even so, my conviction about the forced use of psychiatric medication was now being challenged by Meg's behavior when she was caught up in a manic tailspin.

"What if she really is crazy?" I thought.

Still, intellectually, I knew this couldn't possibly be a coincidence. My sister was furious with me for influencing Meg and claimed I had brainwashed her by equating her experience to mine. She later typed the following in an angry e-mail to our mother:

THIS IS A PART OF HER ILLNESS THAT WILL BECOME FURTHER IMBEDDED IN HER BRAIN IF NOT TREATED AND THEN WILL BECOME EVEN MORE DIFFICULT TO TREAT OVER TIME!!!! Oh, her attitude has improved since she's not MANIC & mean as a snake for now…but she's pretending & I know she is…she thinks that she can pray & think her way out of this & that just isn't so. She needs therapy & I don't have the money…I can't listen to the delusional, twisted thinking anymore because it's about to make me go insane…I would never have imagined how much life could suck in one person's lifetime…I AM MAD AS HELL AT THE SITUATION AND EVERYONE INVOLVED…Oh, but I forgot…Hayley & Peyton & I are really the only ones that are INVOLVED…meanwhile, you two idiots sit around doling out advice when you really don't have to suffer the consequences…MEGAN WILL BE THE ONE TO SUFFER THE CONSEQUENCES ULTIMATELY. WHAT A SHAME…

In early August, during one of Meg's highly agitated states and following a heated argument, Michelle had her arrested on a domestic violence charge. I felt so sorry for Meg. I had spent the previous twenty-four hours attempting to stabilize her. In her condition, I knew jail was the last place she needed to be. Being the only other family member in the area, the court agreed to release Meg to me. So, in search of answers, I started my research for this book after Meg, once again, moved in with my family.

When I went to pick her up from jail she looked terrible. She trembled uncontrollably and rambled incoherently and angrily about how she had been abused. She had been forced to strip naked. She was put into restraints, and she was not given a mat or a blanket to sleep with. She had not slept at all in the cold, concrete holding cell. She was completely manic and talking in loose associations (disconnected thoughts). She was convinced Time Warner was programming her thoughts through the television. She knew she was being spied on through her computer. Everyone was wearing red. It was a sign. Yellow made her nervous and so on. She chain-smoked. Her wrists and arms were badly bruised from the handcuffs and other restraints. Her eyes looked wild, and her pupils were constricted. I'd seen that look plenty before!

We spent the next five days riding out one of the scariest times I could remember since my own psychotic reaction. Meg said she heard command voices that would instruct her to harm herself. She would rapid-cycle, just like I had, from daylight until dark so drastically and so predictably that I started to know at what time to expect the crying jags and then the manic, euphoric moods. I assured Meg this was a drug reaction and she was not schizophrenic. With time and faith, she would heal. She desperately clung to that promise. I also assured her I would always be there for her. It was a promise I would regret because I could not fulfill it. Following a particularly nasty verbal attack on my husband in which she accused him of being the devil, Meg was asked to leave again. She had nowhere to go except back to her mother, a place where she definitely knew, because of being told so repeatedly, she was not wanted.

Meg attempted to withdraw from all of her medications by herself. She even quit smoking. By the time I knew about the severe repercussions of sudden withdrawal from SSRI antidepressants, it was too late. She had been off the drugs for several weeks and could not be reintroduced without additional risk. She suffered horribly debilitating depression and social anxiety. Some days, it was all she could do to get out of bed.

Meg visited a nutritionist and started walking in an attempt to detoxify her body. She wrote and sketched in her journal. She was unable to concentrate well enough to read much. We took drives down to the lake, and would sit listening to CDs and discussing my latest discoveries in research. Still, she and Michelle continued to violently argue. On more than one occasion, the police were called again to the house. Michelle started drinking regularly, and this further upset Meg. She obsessed about the welfare of her younger sisters, Peyton and Hayley. The stress of it all was starting to wear negatively on me again. Plus, I felt my own energy reserves depleting. Out of self-preservation, I tried distancing myself. It is another thing I would live to regret.

Meg had called me early in the morning the day before her suicide. She left a message for me to call her back. When I tried later that morning, the phone had been disconnected. My sister had not paid the bill. I thought Meg might stop in after she picked up her sisters from school. (Their elementary school was right up the street from my house.) She didn't. I thought about driving over to check on her that evening, but I was exhausted. Quite frankly, I was also upset with my sister about the e-mail she had sent that berated my mother and me. So, out of fear of an encounter with my sister, I waited until the next day when I knew Michelle would be at work. I never saw Meg again. My husband and I were en route to the house to check on her when the police called my cell phone. I nearly fainted when they told me Meg had died. A part of me died too. If only I had gone sooner…

The night before Meg ended her life, she and her mother had been arguing. Meg was given an ultimatum: she would have to go back on the drugs or leave. Michelle could not handle Meg's constant dysphoric mood or inability to function socially. Meg still couldn't make a simple trip to Wal-Mart without feeling paranoid and uncomfortable. And here she was faced with the possibility of starting the whole fiasco over again.

This happened even though I had discussed everything I was uncovering in relation to the SSRI category of antidepressants with her and my sister; even though they knew I had experienced the same kind of thing. This occurred even though I had been thoroughly educated on the subject matter and had left my job to do full-time research and write a book about the pharmaceutical cover-ups involved in a number of blockbuster drugs released in the past decade; even though I had expressed a real sense of urgency to alert others. Still, I had only identified the problem. I didn't know how to fix it. I knew Meg's recovery would take time, but I couldn't offer any guarantees or immediate solutions. It appeared the doctors could.

Meg knew I couldn't save her. In spite of all my knowledge and experience, few people were listening to me. This was proven by the fact that my sister was on her way home to forcibly take Meg to the psychiatrist and have her placed on medication again. Why? Because that's what she had been advised to do. Instead, when Michelle arrived at the house, she encountered the police and victim's services. Meg was already gone. Ultimately, *she* would have the final word.

Emotional Anesthesia: Sedating Our Psychic Pain

We hadn't even absorbed the tragedy of Meg's passing yet. All of us were hovered around the fireplace in my family room that evening, including my mother and father; my sister and her friend, Mark; Michelle's ex-husband, Scott; my nieces, Peyton and Hayley; and my husband and I. We sat engulfed in an awkward silence. Nobody really knew what to say. The pain was so acute. Our emotions were so raw and guarded around one another. So, the most inappropriate thing that could have been said was the next topic of conversation. I had to nearly bite a hole through my tongue in order to avoid overreacting.

My sister's friend retrieved two prescription bottles from his coat pocket and explained he had called a doctor friend to get a couple of things to "help Michelle get through this." There were two prescriptions: one for Ativan and one for Xanax. Then he jokingly gestured, extending his hand as though offering everyone around the room.

"Pills anyone? Okay, pills for everybody!" he said with a chuckle as he shook one of the bottles to rattle its contents.

Did he know about the drug reaction Meg had? Did he have any idea what Michelle's history with drug and alcohol dependence had done to her family or her health? Did he know how she would respond to a reintroduction to short-acting benzodiazepines after her adverse withdrawal reactions to Prozac? Did he know about the tremendous addiction potential and withdrawal symptoms associated with these drugs?

That was all my family needed right now, to have another drug tragedy to deal with! Also, that was the last thing my nieces needed, something else to remove their mother emotionally so that she would not be available to comfort or support them in their grief. But, because I felt so paralyzed and so defeated by the battle at that point, I watched in silence as he handed my sister the equivalent of a loaded gun. I simply waited until later to approach my former brother-in-law and ask him to lift them from her purse before the evening was out. I know Mark's intentions were good, but I cannot help but apply the old adage here: "The road to hell is paved with good intentions."

3

A Case against the Antidepressants: Prescription for Disaster

"Whatever is hidden will be brought out into the open and whatever is covered up, will be uncovered."

—(Mark 4:22)

It is estimated that one out of every six Americans has taken an antidepressant drug. Antidepressants are prescribed for back pain, premenstrual syndrome (PMS), hot flashes, post-traumatic stress disorder (PTSD), depression, chronic pain, weight loss, muscle pain, anxiety, obsessive-compulsive disorder (OCD), smoking cessation, and sleep disturbance, to name just a few. Antidepressants were the best-selling class of drugs between 1999 and 2001 and ranked third in 2002 and 2003 behind cholesterol-lowering statins and acid-suppressing drugs. In 2003, manufacturers sold $19.5 billion of antidepressants boasting a 10 percent year-over-year sales growth ("IMS Reports 9 Percent Constant Dollar Growth in '03 Global Pharma Sales").

The cover-ups, misrepresentation of data, false advertising, and biased clinical research associated with the SSRI antidepressant drugs is staggering. I was shocked to learn of a network of SSRI survivors across the nation, who have either experienced the horror of an adverse reaction themselves or a loved one's death as a result of these drugs. The side effects reported with antidepressant use include mood swings, lack of emotion, vivid and violent dreams, altered personality, racing thoughts, restlessness, inability to sit still, unusual energy surges, inability to recognize reality, silly or giddy behavior, paranoia, blank staring, hyperactivity, aggression, self-destructive behavior, violence, suicidal thoughts and attempts, mania, and psychosis (Ko).

History reminds us that it took twenty years after Eli Lilly and Parke-Davis introduced LSD and PCP in the United States before the government declared them illegal. Eli Lilly first produced and marketed LSD in the 1950s as an aid to psychoanalysis, a cure for alcoholism, and a way to clear up mental disorders.

19

Parke-Davis promoted angel dust or PCP as an analgesic and anesthesia. Of course, Dr. Sigmund Freud was one of the strongest supporters of the medicinal use of cocaine in psychiatry before he became addicted. Interestingly, all of these drugs act on the brain by increasing serotonin levels. It would be fair to conclude that psychiatry has given us some of the most addictive, destructive drugs ever recorded in history. Is history repeating itself?

Several of the leading authorities in psychiatry have come forward to denounce the excessive use of the SSRIs and alert people to the similarities in their clinical uses and side effects to the neuroleptic drugs. Neurological side effects seen with the serotonin-boosters and other dangers not commonly acknowledged by their manufacturers now litter psychiatric literature and case studies.

Depending on its severity, neurologically-driven agitation can be quite dangerous. This was soon to be discovered when large numbers of children, who had no previous indication of being suicidal, began taking their lives after only brief exposure to these drugs. If a patient has not been warned about this potential side effect and confuses it with the deterioration of his or her own emotional and mental state, it can produce abject terror and precipitate psychosis and suicidal tendencies.

It was the staggering increase in drug-related suicide that eventually resulted in the FDA's requirement for manufacturers to place a black box warning on all antidepressants regarding this increased risk in children and adolescents. However, even that didn't happen until September 2004, and it required two congressional inquiries. (The first of which took place three years earlier in 2001!) Manufacturers fought vehemently against these warnings and claimed more harm than good could result if patients declined treatment. They have continued to point to the disease being treated as the cause of suicide rather than the drugs they produce.

In an article appearing in the *Journal of Clinical Psychiatry* in 1989, only two years after the release of Prozac, doctors were already starting to report drug-induced neurological agitation. The article claimed the agitation was "clinically indistinguishable" from that caused by neuroleptic drugs. It declared neurologically driven agitation to be a common side effect of the drug and estimated to occur in ten to twenty-five percent of patients. Similar reports connected with Zoloft, Paxil, and Luvox started to appear in the literature once they were introduced (Glenmullen 47).

In 1990, a Harvard researcher, Dr. Martin Teicher, and two associates, Carol Clod and Jonathan Cole, published an article in the *American Journal of Psychia-*

try that discussed six cases in which patients on Prozac had become intensely pre-occupied with ideas of suicide. Subsequently, Dr. Teicher was discredited and portrayed as an alarmist in the scientific community.

That same year, another group of Harvard researchers made an alarming disclosure in the *American Journal of Psychiatry*. This Prozac clinical trial involved depressed adolescents, and it was conducted by the University of South Carolina. The study was stopped abruptly because of the "emergence of intense violent suicidal and/or homicidal ideation in five patients" (Breggin, *Talking Back to Prozac*, 163).

In March 1991, yet another group of researchers at the Yale University School of Medicine published a report on the "Emergence of Self-Destructive Phenomena in Children and Adolescents during Fluoxetine Treatment." In the report, the authors stated that:

> Self-injurious ideation or behavior appeared de novo [for the first time] or intensified in six of forty-seven patients being treated with Prozac for obsessive-compulsive disorder. Four of the cases required hospitalization and three required restraints, seclusion, or one-to-one nursing care (Breggin, *Talking Back to Prozac*, 165).

In 1997, Dr. David Healy, former secretary of the British Association for Psychopharmacology and author of *Let Them Eat Prozac*, conducted an antidepressant clinical trial on a group of healthy volunteers in North Wales. The group consisted of eleven women and nine men between the ages of twenty-seven and fifty-two. All were senior and junior nurses and consulting or training psychiatrists. The study was a comparison between the antidepressants Zoloft (sertraline) and Edronax (reboxetine). It was designed to asses the "better than well" phenomenon described by some Prozac users. It should be noted that Edronax is a SNRI (selective norepinephrine reuptake inhibitor) drug that has not been approved for use in the United States.

Shortly into the study, Dr. Healy noticed an unusual number of side effects not listed for either drug. After breaking the blind, Healy noted:

> 2/3 of the group felt significantly worse on one of the two drugs—not simply by virtue of inconvenient side effects, such as difficulties in passing water [urination], but in terms of being depressed or disturbed or in some other way realizing this was not a drug for them. The implication was there was a very high chance, perhaps approaching fifty-fifty, that primary-care physi-

cians could put their patients on a pill unsuitable for them (Healy, *Let Them Eat Prozac*, 180-181).

Two of the patients in the study group became suicidal. Healy recounts this startling development of events with one participant named Joanna:

...she looked almost shrunken, worried, and nervous. She withdrew from interactions with others. She began impulsively spending money and doing other things she was reluctant to tell. She might begin to cry for no reason. Her moods swung from gloom to doom in a matter of minutes, so much that a number of people described her as almost manic. She had repeated dreams of slitting her throat and bleeding to death in bed beside her mate (Healy, *Let Them Eat Prozac*, 182-183).

Joanna's nightmare would culminate one night as she struggled with her sanity and the overwhelming impulse to throw herself in front of a car or a train. She was on her way out the door to kill herself when the phone rang, disrupting her hypnotic state and saving her life (Healy, *Let Them Eat Prozac*, 183–184).

Dr. Healy was alarmed that his trial had picked up an effect like suicide in such a small group of totally normal people. The second participant that became suicidal was haunted by the theme of hanging. This theme is common to many SSRI-related suicides. Both participants were females who had shown "lower than average traces of any kind of depressive thinking" prior to drug treatment. It was later discovered that both were taking Zoloft.

According to Dr. Healy, the women remained "greatly disturbed several months later; seriously questioning the stability of their own personalities." This struck him as "ludicrous." However, he said he had great difficulty persuading them it had been the drug and only the drug. Their view of themselves had been shaken. The experience had "at least a medium-term impact on both women's self-esteem" (Healy, *Let Them Eat Prozac*, 185–187).

By 1999, the FDA had received 2,000 reports of suicide by Prozac users. Of which, about twenty-five percent could be linked to akathisia and agitation reactions. According to the FDA's own estimates, it only receives reports on approximately one to ten percent of all adverse reactions. That would imply that as many as 50,000 akathisia-related suicides could be attributed to Prozac alone. The total estimate for the entire SSRI class of drugs would, of course, be much higher (DeGrandpre).

So, if there is so much information available about these life-threatening, adverse reactions and if it has been in the literature since the introduction of the SSRIs, why are so many doctors uninformed about it? In defense of private practicing physicians who often work twelve-to fourteen-hour days, are required to do ever-increasing amounts of administrative work, and see large patient loads, there really is little leisure time for reading. I often saw desktops laden with journals and other unopened mail. If it suits their cause, pharmaceutical reps may point out the latest studies about a drug. If it does not, they may go undiscovered by the doctor for some time.

Unfortunately, doctors still frequently mistake akathisia symptoms for agitated depression. In which case, the common rationale is to increase the blood levels more rapidly by upping the dose. So, instead of discontinuing the drug, the dosage is increased. The agitation is then magnified, which is a combination for disaster.

Part of the problem that exists here is embedded in the highly dynamic patient-doctor relationship. The doctor assumes an authoritative position, making it more difficult for the patient to stop taking a drug in the case of adverse reactions. When things go wrong in the case of SSRIs, the situation can escalate very rapidly. The dynamics of this crisis are comparable to a hostage situation. The doctor, who has probably unwittingly trapped the patient, becomes the only way out. The patient may be too frightened to even question—much less go against—what the doctor has advised. When the doctor instructs the patient to continue taking the medication or increase the dose when the patient is going mad, it takes an extremely brave person to do the opposite (Healy, *Let Them Eat Prozac*, 274).

Discontinuation Syndrome: A Nice Name for Withdrawal

Patients using antidepressants are at risk for suicidal ideation and behavior both while using the drug as well as in the months following discontinuation of the drug. The new FDA warnings specifically address the need to monitor this risk while increasing or decreasing the dose. Therefore, it is imperative that patients wanting to discontinue or taper off the dose of their medication do so under a doctor's supervision. The first couple of months are generally the riskiest; however, depending on the length of time the antidepressant has been used, it can take several months to successfully discontinue treatment ("Dr. Glenmullen's Q & A: Antidepressant Side Effects").

Effexor, the drug Meg took for more than eight months and stopped abruptly, is cited as one of the worst antidepressants in terms of causing severe withdrawal reactions, especially the increased risk for suicide. In fact, in August 2003, Wyeth, the drug's manufacturer, issued a warning letter to doctors because it was concerned about clinical trial evidence linking Effexor to suicidal thoughts in young patients. In that letter, the company announced to practitioners that it would be adding the following statement to the precautions section of the Effexor label: "In pediatric clinical trials, there were increased reports of hostility and, especially in Major Depressive Disorder, suicide-related adverse events such as suicidal ideation and self-harm." Subsequently, the FDA asked Wyeth to remove its precaution and replace it with the more generic *class labeling*. An FDA spokesperson said the agency had asked Wyeth to change the precaution because the statement represented a discrepancy with the FDA-approved warning required on all antidepressants in March 2004. That warning states that "it has not been concluded that these drugs cause worsening depression or suicidality."

Now, almost a year later, a new FDA analysis appears to validate Wyeth's original concern. Of the six drugs that were compared in the analysis, the results of the three Wyeth clinical trials for Effexor showed that young patients on the drug were nearly five times as likely to have suicidal thoughts or behavior as those on placebo. When just the data of the two trials on depression were analyzed, suicidal tendencies were 8.8 times as likely in the young patients taking Effexor (Wilde Mathews).

Some statistics from studies of patients affected by withdrawal when they stopped taking their antidepressants cold turkey include seventy-eight percent of Effexor patients, sixty-six percent of Paxil patients, sixty percent of Zoloft patients, and fourteen percent of Prozac patients. Depending on how quickly the drug washes out of the body, withdrawal reactions can range from mild to severe ("Dr. Glenmullen's Q & A: Antidepressant Side Effects"). Meg had complained of debilitating depression, social phobia, and electrical shock waves that ran through her brain, which her mother thought was a psychotic delusion.

Symptoms of SSRI and SNRI antidepressant withdrawal can include, but are not limited to, suicide, impulsivity, aggression, anxiety, depression, crying spells, insomnia, dizziness, vertigo, nausea, vomiting, headaches, tremors, and electric "zap" sensations in the brain. Symptoms can be so severe that patients cannot get out of bed or work. In these cases, the dosage should be tapered off more slowly. The patient should also allow additional time before completely discontinuing the drug (Dr. Glenmullen's Q & A: Antidepressant Side Effects").

Typical Concerns Raised by the Atypical Antidepressants

One atypical antidepressant that has become fairly popular for treating depression as well as smoking cessation is Wellbutrin (buproprion). In fact, Wellbutrin's twin, Zyban, was introduced specifically to capture the market for the latter indication and extend the patent on buproprion. Wellbutrin blocks the neurotransmitter dopamine rather than serotonin. The risk of seizure with Wellbutrin has been found to be four times greater than with other antidepressants. The danger increases to tenfold at twice the normal daily dose of 300 milligrams. People who have had head injury, brain and spinal tumors, or previous seizures are at the greatest risk. Seizures may also be precipitated by an abrupt increase in the dosage.

Some patients experience central nervous system effects that produce a very unpleasant hypersensitivity. Agitation, anxiety, and insomnia are often reported at the beginning of Wellbutrin therapy. The simultaneous use of a tricyclic antidepressant can further increase the risk of seizure.

Serzone, another atypical antidepressant that was launched in 1994 and is manufactured by Bristol-Myers Squibb (BMS), was voluntarily withdrawn from the Canadian market because of reports of liver injury late in 2003. Earlier in 2003, BMS had also voluntarily pulled the drug from markets in Europe, Spain, and Turkey. Finally, citing commercial reasons, BMS stopped shipment of Serzone in the United States on June 14, 2004. Currently, there is a class action suit for Serzone injuries in the United States. Litigants in the case cite severe side effects including liver impairment, liver failure, and death resulting from Serzone use. (Fortunately, I was never required to sell Serzone when I worked for BMS because I was in the cardiovascular division.)

The Depression Epidemic

The World Health Organization has projected that depression will be the second-leading cause of disability in the world by 2020, following heart disease. Depression impacts millions of Americans annually, specifically an estimated ten percent of the population at any given time. Women experience depression twice as often as men do. Many circumstances can predispose an individual to depression, including loss of a parent, emotional neglect, or trauma experienced in childhood or stressful life experiences in general, for example, death, divorce, job loss, or other financial stress. A genetic link is also suggested because depression frequently runs in families.

Depression and anxiety can manifest simultaneously in some people, and these diseases share many common symptoms (for example, irritability, fatigue, sleep disturbance, ruminating thoughts, appetite disruption, cognitive difficulties, and guilt feelings). Although some depression can be attributed to medical conditions such as thyroid disease or cancer, the majority of mild to moderate depression is primarily thought to have a psychological origin. Depression is defined by some psychologists as "anger turned inward." These mild to moderate depressions are the main diagnoses for which antidepressant drugs are most frequently prescribed and the conditions for which the SSRIs have proven to be least effective.

However, there are more serious types of depression such as major clinical depression. This depression runs a definite course of time (that is, it has a beginning, middle, and an end to each episode), whereas, dysthymia is a chronic type of depression that generally lasts more than two years. Manic-depressive (bipolar) disorder, on the other hand, is a little more difficult to define. Mild to extreme euphoria and grandiosity can alternate with moderate to radically low depressive states. Their course and severity are both completely unpredictable. There are three major types of bipolar disorders: bipolar I, bipolar II, and cyclothymia. (Refer to the glossary for definitions.)

The Biogenic Amine Deficiency Theory of Depression

Nearly all of the antidepressants currently being marketed or in various stages of development in pharmaceutical pipelines are based on the biogenic amine deficiency theory. This theory assumes depression is caused by some deficiency in either the neurotransmitter serotonin or norepinephrine activity in the brain. Translated loosely, this means there is a chemical imbalance in the brain.

I love the current Zoloft commercial with the little, bouncing, happy face explaining depression may be attributed to a chemical imbalance in the brain and Zoloft corrects that imbalance. That simply is not so! The biochemical imbalance speculation is just that, speculation presented by industry as a scientific truth.

Most of our biochemical research on emotional states addresses only three or four of the more than 100 neurotransmitters now estimated to be present in the brain. The newest antidepressant drugs still only act on two or three neurotransmitters, even though they are touted as having more specific receptor targets than the older drugs (Valenstein 109–110).

The fact is there is absolutely no convincing evidence that most depressed people have low levels of biogenic amine activity. Reputable researchers working in the psychopharmacology field recognize the inadequacy of this theory and are trying to come up with alternative theories. Moreover, there is no reason to assume any biochemical deficiency is the cause of any mental disorder. Low serotonin levels are associated with a variety of psychological disorders and cannot be used to predict or identify any specific problem. Because we know stress can affect brain chemistry, it is entirely plausible that emotions are responsible for the low serotonin and norepinephrine levels, rather than the other way around (WORLD Magazine). The irony of all this is that the only known biochemical imbalance found in the brains of nearly all mental patients has been caused by the patient's psychiatric treatments (Breggin, *Talking Back to Prozac*, 39).

A less popular but more accurate theory is the biopsychosocial model. This model suggests that three areas of life interact to create psychological problems, including depression: 1) Our biology as determined by our genes, brain chemistry, medical conditions and drugs; 2) the individual collection of feelings, desires, thoughts, and behaviors that comprise our own unique psychology; and 3) the events and people in our social experience that shape our life (Drummond 16).

Minimal Efficacy—Mega Risk

Not only does a tremendous amount of evidence suggest these drugs are harmful to large numbers of people, there is also inadequate scientific evidence to support they are any more effective than the older, less expensive antidepressants.

A vigilant research group in the United States utilized the Freedom of Information Act (FOIA) to obtain all of the studies (both published and unpublished) the FDA had used in their determination to approve seven of the newer antidepressants between 1987 and 1997. They included studies done on Prozac, Zoloft, Paxil, Effexor, Serzone, Remeron, and Wellbutrin SR. After reviewing all of the results from the individual manufacturers' pivotal studies, the researchers concluded the newer antidepressants were "no more effective than the older tricyclic antidepressants." In fact, the newer drugs were not found to be even ten percent more effective than placebos:

> Symptoms of depression improved by 30.9 percent in the people who took the placebos; by 40.7 percent in the people who took the newer antidepressants; and by 41.7 percent in people who took the older antidepressants.

For people with mild to moderate depression, "nine out of ten studies showed that the new drugs were no more effective than placebos" (Abramson 116).

However, because of the great marketing hype surrounding the SSRIs, one of them, Prozac, now has the distinguished honor of having more adverse effects submitted to the FDA than any other drug in history. More than 40,000 adverse reactions were reported in its first ten years on the market. No other drug even comes close (Breggin and Cohen 67).

There have been multiple reports of fraudulent clinical testing, forgery, bribery, racketeering, and endangering patients in the testing of psychiatric drugs. Two big scandals rocked clinical research in 1993, which was the same year Warner Brothers released its mega hit, *The Fugitive*, starring Harrison Ford. One scandal involved the National Institutes of Health (NIH) and Eli Lilly's clinical trials of an anti-hepatitis drug named Fialuridine. Test subjects suddenly started to drop dead of liver failure (just like the story in *The Fugitive*). The study was halted.

Immediately following that scandal, a renowned child psychiatrist and teen suicide expert, Dr. Barry Garfinkel, was found guilty of two counts of mail fraud and three counts of filing false statements. He would later serve six months in a halfway house and six months under house arrest and pay $210,000 in fines and restitution. Why? In 1989, while conducting a study of the antidepressant Anafranil (clomipramine) at the University of Minnesota, Dr. Garfinkel had instructed a study coordinator to "invent data on patient visits that had never taken place—eye examinations and physicals that were supposed to be done to make sure the drug wasn't harming the test subjects." It had taken the case four years to come to court (Fried 77–78).

In 1997, another case hit the news involving the chairman of the department of psychiatry at the Medical College of Georgia and one of its professors. Richard Borison and Bruce Diamond were convicted on 172 counts and were each fined $125,000. However, the crime for which they would serve time was not to be fraudulent clinical testing. It would be for stealing from the college. Borison and Diamond were ordered by the court to pay $4.26 million and $1.1 million respectively to the college. Borison was sentenced to fifteen years in prison. Diamond was sentenced to five years. These two psychopharmacologists were connected with the clinical testing of psychiatric drugs with twenty different companies for more than a decade. The companies included Eli Lilly, Janssen, Zeneca, Sandoz, Glaxo, Abbott, Pfizer, and Hoechst Marion Roussel. Borison and Diamond were reported to have secured 160 contracts from drug companies and made over $10 million on drug research during that time (Whitaker 269).

In 1998, the Minnesota Board of Medical Practice suspended the license of another prominent psychiatric researcher, Dr. Frank Abuzzahab, the past president of the Minnesota Psychiatric Society and the chairman of its ethics committee, who was found "guilty of recklessly entering patients into psychiatric drug studies, falsifying their records, and fabricating positive drug responses." Dr. Abuzzahab was one of the lead investigators in a clinical trial Eli Lilly submitted to the FDA for its approval of Prozac (Glenmullen, *Prozac Backlash*, 209).

In an analysis of more than eighty clinical studies of the newer antidepressants, the Agency for Health Care Policy and Research in the Department of Health and Human Services found that, overall, half of the patients did not respond to the drugs. For those who did, sixty-four percent of the benefit was attributed to placebo effect. Why were placebos so effective in these studies? People with mild to moderate depression are very responsive to attention and suggestion. Many patients come to these clinical studies with hope for recovery. They establish supportive relationships with interviewers and caretakers because they are evaluated and monitored frequently. These circumstances alone may be all some people need to work through their depressive episode (Glenmullen, *Prozac Backlash*, 208).

Children are even more susceptible to suggestion than adults. That is why study after study has shown antidepressants to be no more effective in children than placebos. A review was published in the *Journal of Nervous and Mental Disease* in 1996 in which the authors concluded, "The evidence is unanimous that antidepressants are no more effective than placebos in children with symptoms of depression." They then cited several other reviewers that had come to the same conclusion (Glenmullen, *Prozac Backlash*, 208).

A blatant example of the misrepresentation of the SSRIs efficacy in children and adolescents is provided by the Paxil studies for the treatment of depressed adolescents. GlaxoSmithKline published a study in 2001 that showed "depressed adolescents were significantly more likely to improve when treated with Paxil than when treated with a placebo." In May 2003, British drug authorities acquired all nine studies that were done on Paxil for the treatment of adolescents under the age of eighteen. This included the one published study and eight unpublished studies. A compilation of this data showed a very different picture than the published article had represented. "The patients were no less depressed after taking Paxil than after taking placebos, and the incidence of emotional lability (including suicidal thoughts) was twice as high (3.2 percent versus 1.5 percent)." This prompted the United Kingdom Medicines and Healthcare Products Regulatory Agency to advise doctors against prescribing Paxil for patients under the age of eighteen (Abramson 117).

On January 3, 2004, Prozac became the only SSRI currently approved for use in depressed children ages seven to seventeen. However, the study Eli Lilly used to gain that additional indication also raises questions upon closer inspection. According to Vera Sharav of the Alliance for Human Research Protection, "At least two of the 48 children treated with Prozac in the National Institute of Mental Health (NIMH)-sponsored trial [had] attempted suicide..." However, in the single published report of this trial that appeared in *Archives of General Psychiatry*, there is no mention of any children having attempted suicide. Instead, the published report states: "Side effects, as a reason for discontinuation, were minimal, affecting only 4 patients who were receiving Prozac." In 2001, FDA reviewers looked at three pooled Prozac pediatric trials and found that "22 children dropped out because of adverse reactions in the Prozac-treated group compared to five in the placebo groups." The review also noted there were three suicide attempts among the Prozac group versus one in the placebo group. "Further-more, six of the Prozac-treated children, but none on placebo, developed mania or hypomania" (Gardner, F).

The bottom line is, tucked away and unavailable to the public eye without someone going to great lengths to obtain all the data, is the indisputable, but well-hidden, fact that not only are these drugs ineffective, but the "actual rate of death from suicide is higher in patients who take the new antidepressants than in those who take the older tricyclics," or who receive no treatment at all. That's right! The statistical results of all the published and unpublished data revealed, out of every 1000 persons with depression that were treated with one of the new antidepressant drugs, 4.6 more committed suicide each year than would have if they had not received any treatment at all (Abramson 116).

Keep in mind, in the studies that won the SSRIs initial FDA approval, seri-ously depressed patients, anyone suicidal, those with manic/depression, children, and the elderly were typically excluded. These drugs are currently prescribed like candy to all of these groups. Often, as you will see, it is with dire consequences.

4

A "Chill Pill" to Kill

"A man's spirit sustains him in sickness but a crushed spirit who can bear?"

—(Proverbs 18:14)

On December 9, 2004, exactly one week following Megan's suicide, *Primetime Live* broadcast an exposé on the dangers of antidepressants. Under the circumstances, it was a bone-chilling report. I could barely stand to listen to the 9-1-1 calls played in the broadcast. Family members begged for help sounding terrified and desperate as their children tried to kill themselves. A ten-year-old girl was heard begging and screaming repeatedly, "I want to die! I want to die!" in the background ("Drug Company Investigation"). The hair literally stood on the back of my neck. If only my sister had seen this report a week earlier, maybe things would have turned out differently. There were so many of these "if only" moments to reflect on.

A staggering number of cases are pending against pharmaceutical manufacturers of antidepressants as well as the doctors who prescribed them. By 1994, there were 160 cases against Prozac alone. Homicide and suicide cases, where behavior is attributed to adverse drug reactions, continue to pile up on court dockets. In fact, some have been highly publicized. Many others have been settled and given gag orders as terms of the settlement. Still others will remain tied up in litigation for years.

While we look at a few of the shattered lives left in the wake of the SSRIs, see if you can identify some of the symptoms that would signify an adverse SSRI reaction in the following patient case studies. What may seem like isolated incidents appear to form a pattern when the stories are grouped together. Keep in mind, in a review of the media and survivor group reports on violence, violence and murder were found to be "quite rare among depressed patients." Therefore, it is impossible to attribute the following horrible events to depression, the disease, itself (Breggin, *Talking Back to Prozac*, 159).

31

The Pittman Trial

A tragic case that recently made major headlines from South Carolina involved a young boy named Christopher (Chris) Pittman. Chris was sentenced to thirty years in prison after being found guilty of shotgunning his grandparents to death and setting their house on fire. The murders occurred just weeks after Chris was started on the antidepressant Zoloft. He had previously been on Paxil. Only days before the murders, Pittman's psychiatrist had doubled the dose of his medication. Chris was twelve years old at the time. At five feet, one inch tall, he only weighed ninety-seven pounds. The forensic psychologist and other experts retained by Pittman's attorney claimed Chris' actions were definitely triggered by an adverse drug reaction. Of course, Pfizer, the manufacturer of Zoloft, refuted this possibility. Its representative, Dr. Steve Romano, testified the causal link between Zoloft use and aggression/suicide could not be substantiated. He further stated, in early February, the FDA had issued "a new label for Zoloft that deleted any references to a causal link between antidepressants and an increase in aggression" (Springer).

CBS profiled this case in a *48 Hours* piece, "Prescription for Murder," that aired on April 16, 2005, following Christopher's conviction. I sat numbly watching as the report revealed Chris' experience of many of the adverse reactions I have addressed here. On the day of the murders, Chris had been disciplined by his grandparents. Chris had gotten into a fight with a much younger student on the school bus, and he was also reported to have been fidgeting and kicking the piano bench in church earlier that evening. Both incidents were obvious signs of agitation. Chris' sister reported Chris had been almost manic at Thanksgiving. She said he was talking rapidly and had started several sentences without finishing them, as though his thoughts were racing faster than he could express them. Chris had also complained to an aunt that he did not like the drug he was taking because it made him "feel like [his] skin [was] crawling." When questioned by the interviewer if he knew what he was doing at the time of the murders, Chris said he felt like he was "watching a movie" and was unable to control his actions or his intense feelings of anger and agitation. Chris said he had heard a voice in his head telling him to "kill," and it just kept getting louder.

The prosecutors in the case pointed to the emotional blunting Chris exhibited after he was apprehended in order to portray him as a cold-blooded, premeditated killer with no remorse whatsoever for his actions. However, family members and clergy painted quite a different picture. They described Chris as a shy, introverted little boy who dearly loved his grandparents. In fact, he had run away from his father's home in Florida because he wanted to live with them. This side of the story also revealed a troubled child that had been abandoned by his mother and shuffled back and forth between his grandparents' home in South Carolina and his father's home in Florida. His father had been married and divorced three times. It was obvious Chris had suffered tremendous loss.

When one member of the jury was questioned about the guilty verdict, he said he and others simply couldn't believe a drug could cause somebody to kill.

"A million people take it every day," he said." Why would he be the only one who reacts like this?"

That is a good question. Unfortunately, Chris Pittman *isn't* the only one to react this way!

Because he was tried as an adult for a crime he committed at the age of twelve, Chris Pittman will not be eligible for parole until he is forty-two years old, even though several experts testified Pittman acted under the influence of toxic, mind-altering drugs he was given by his doctor. Where is the justice in that? First, this child and his family were victimized by the health care system. Then they were victimized, again, by the legal system. Apparently, Pfizer could afford a better legal defense than Chris Pittman. The closing screen of this documentary was Pfizer's written disclaimer that "Zoloft has not been proven to cause homicidal tendencies" ("Prescription for Murder").

(Please note that no offense is intended to Andy Vickery, the Houston attorney who defended Pittman. He provided his service free of charge, and he obviously had Chris' best interests at heart. Unfortunately, litigation of this nature is very costly. Moreover, a pharmaceutical company's financial and legal resources are unlimited. It has been my personal experience that pharmaceutical companies will do anything in order to protect their financial interests.)

The Hawkins Case

In the summer of 2001, a Supreme Court judge in Australia delivered a verdict clearly finding that David Hawkins, a seventy-three-year-old man who had murdered his wife the day after going on Zoloft and who also had a prior history of an adverse reaction to Zoloft, would not have committed the act if he had not been on the drug (Healy, *Let Them Eat Prozac*, 219). After strangling his wife, Mr. Hawkins was reported to have said:

> I have killed my wife…I got tablets from the doctor yesterday and I think they were too strong. I went, I went absolutely wild. I don't know. I was mad. I can't say any more…I have got to go. I am heading out and I am

going to get rid of myself. Nobody, nobody can help me now. Nobody can help me now. Look I've got to go. I'm shaking here. I can't wait. I can't stop (Tracy 2001).

The Johnston Case

In 2001, Jay Johnston was awarded $3 million following an antidepressant negligence suit. Johnston, a strapping, seventeen-year-old, high-school jock from Oregon, tried committing suicide after being prescribed Zoloft, Ritalin, and Prozac. In 1996, Johnston had sought treatment for depression from his family doctor. The doctor first prescribed Zoloft and Ritalin. Johnston claimed to have attempted suicide. His doctor initially increased the medication, but she ultimately switched him to Prozac. In the spring of 1997, following arguments with his mother and a friend, Johnston put a shotgun to his chin and made another attempt to end his life. He survived the blast, but he is now grossly disfigured. His doctor filed an appeal (Nielsen).

The Tobin Case

In June 2001, a Wyoming jury ordered GlaxoSmithKline to pay several million dollars to the family of Donald Schell. Schell was a sixty-year-old man who murdered his wife, daughter, and granddaughter before he killed himself, two days after starting on the company's drug, Paxil (paroxetine).

Schell had a history of problems with his nerves, primarily stress related to work and bereavements. He had previously had an adverse reaction to Prozac in 1990. As noted by his previous doctor, Prozac had made Schell become tense, anxious, and jittery despite several antidotes (Inderal, Ativan and Desyrel) given to him in order to combat these symptoms.

Donald Schell had been married to his wife, Rita for thirty-seven years. They had two children named Michael and Deborah. Nine months earlier, Deborah had given birth to the Schell's first grandchild, and she had brought the baby from Billings to visit for a few days in February 1998.

Also in February 1998, Schell began complaining about difficulties in sleeping, so he and his wife visited a primary care physician. The doctor did a thorough examination, which included rating scales that indicated Mr. Schell's main complaint to be poor sleep. The ratings also revealed Mr. Schell felt hopeful about the future and thought well of himself. Schell's doctor diagnosed an anxiety state and prescribed Paxil. Unaware of Schell's previous negative response to Prozac, he did not prescribe any covering antidotes for side effects such as agitation. Forty-eight hours later, Donald Schell put three bullets from two different guns through Rita's head and then through Deborah and Alyssa's heads before shooting and killing himself.

On June 6, 2001, the Wyoming jury awarded for damages "four times greater than the biggest previous award in Wyoming—a first-ever verdict against a pharmaceutical company for a psychiatric side effect of a psychotropic drug" (Healy, *Let Them Eat Prozac*, 222). Paxil's manufacturer was ordered to pay $6.4 million after some very damaging company records were exposed in the trial. Several things were revealed that GlaxoSmithKline had not disclosed. For example, in the 1980s, it was discovered that healthy volunteers on Paxil were suffering withdrawal symptoms after discontinuation with only a couple weeks of use. In a trial performed with healthy company employees that had not previously exhibited depressive symptoms, as many as eighty-five percent suffered agitation, abnormal dreams, insomnia, and so forth. An average of fifty percent of volunteers exhibited physical dependence on Paxil. In thirty-four studies performed on healthy volunteers, they found that twenty-five percent had become agitated on Paxil. Some healthy volunteers even became suicidal. One leading investigator made notes documenting his surprise at the large number of problems reported by healthy volunteers (Tracy 2001).

The Miller Case

Matthew Miller was thirteen years old when the sudden changes of puberty and his family's move to a new community caused him to become depressed. Matthew could not seem to penetrate the cliques in his new school. His parents said he complained he felt like an outsider and was angry at everybody. His grades suffered. Matt's teachers administered a set of tests, and Matt fell marginally on the outside range of normal. However, Matt's parents agreed to take him to see a psychiatrist. The psychiatrist diagnosed Matthew as having either a depressive disorder or attention deficit/hyperactivity disorder. He enthusiastically endorsed a "terrific new medication" and urged Matthew's parents to have him try it for "just one week." He told them it would improve Matt's mood and make him feel better about himself. The doctor just happened to be a consultant and speaker for Pfizer (Healy, *Let Them Eat Prozac*, 196).

During the next week, Matt's grandmother noticed Matt was fidgety, "jumping out of his skin." Then, on July 28, 1997, after Matt had taken the last tablet of his one-week trial of Zoloft, he reportedly "got out of bed, went to his closet, and hung himself." His parents were devastated. Matt did not leave a note, and there had been no previous attempts of suicide. Matt had ended his life impulsively. His parents, who were in the next room, never even heard a sound (Ko).

Pfizer fought the case and argued suicide is the second-most common cause of death in thirteen-year-old males. That is true; however, thirteen-year old children don't die very often. One of their experts even argued Matt may have hanged himself by accident in an act of *autoerotic asphyxiation* gone wrong (Healy, *Let Them Eat Prozac*, 197).

The Wesbecker Case

The most convincing evidence of a cover-up involving the litigation with one of these drugs was exposed in the Wesbecker Trial of 1994. It was one of the earlier Prozac cases. Unfortunately, this trial coincided with the O.J. Simpson trial that caused a media frenzy, so it received scant attention in the news at the time. To read a riveting account of this case, John Cornwell wrote about it in *The Power to Harm.*

Five years earlier, Joseph Wesbecker went on a murderous rampage with an AK-47 in Louisville, Kentucky, killing and maiming several of his coworkers. His wrongful death suit became a legal publicity scandal when it ended with a not guilty verdict.

Wesbecker had a poor, difficult childhood, which included time spent in an orphanage. He began working as a printing press operator in his early twenties. He married and had two sons. Economic stress in the 1970s increased pressure on him and other employees at Standard Gravure as fewer employees were expected to produce more work. Wesbecker's marriage dissolved. He started seeing a psychiatrist and was diagnosed with depression. After attempting suicide, Wesbecker was placed on a number of different medications.

In 1988, Wesbecker's psychiatrist prescribed the new wonder drug known as Prozac. Wesbecker stopped taking the drug after only a couple of days claiming it "didn't suit him." He then went on disability in the spring of 1989. His psychiatrist suggested he try Prozac again. A month later, when Wesbecker returned for a follow-up appointment, his psychiatrist found he was agitated and combative. His psychiatrist requested that Wesbecker discontinue the Prozac, but Wesbecker refused. When asked why, Wesbecker claimed it had helped him remember an incident at work in which he had been required to perform fellatio on a foreman while other workers watched.

Several witnesses reported Wesbecker was not himself over the next few days. He was agitated, could not sleep, and paced the floor endlessly. His appearance was slovenly and unkempt. His wife claimed he had gotten up three times to use the bathroom during dinner the night before the murders and he had barely eaten any food.

On September 14, Wesbecker went to the Standard Gravure printing presses with an AK-47 and other guns. He then killed eight people and severely wounded twelve others. He was reported to have walked methodically through the plant firing his weapons. Then he shot himself.

As it turned out, Wesbecker's psychotic delusion in which he alleged sexual abuse is a type of adverse reaction to Prozac. It has since been reported in other settings, and it was also a phenomenon that was found in Eli Lilly's Prozac trials (Healy, *Let Them Eat Prozac*, 64–65).

Later, it was discovered Eli Lilly's attorneys had struck a private deal with the plaintiffs. The defense counsel bartered with the prosecution and promised a substantial financial settlement, regardless of the case's outcome, if they would withhold the submission of critical evidence. All of this was done behind the back of the presiding judge, John Potter.

In 1996, Judge Potter discovered the deception and filed documents demanding Eli Lilly be forced to disclose the secret terms of the settlement they had reached with the plaintiffs. He later told the Kentucky Supreme Court that "Lilly sought to buy not just the verdict, but the court's judgment as well" and further claimed Eli Lilly had widely publicized the not guilty verdict to imply they had "proven in a court of law that Prozac was safe." Judge Potter insisted "a full and open disclosure of the terms of the settlement [was] a necessary public safety issue" (Tracy 2001).

Come to find out, the damaging evidence that was withheld from the jury was information about the Oraflex scandal in the 1980s. Eli Lilly's track record of hiding information from the FDA about liver-related deaths that had occurred in clinical trials with this drug would have established a precedent of Eli Lilly's blatant disregard for public safety and previous misrepresentation of data to regulatory agencies. This backhanded agreement had assisted the defense in winning its not guilty verdict. Therefore, the record was later revised to reflect a settlement. Unfortunately, by that time, the media was no longer interested in the case, and few people were aware of the deception.

The Forsyth Case

William Forsyth retired with his wife of thirty-five years in 1990. They relocated to beautiful Maui, Hawaii. Bill was sixty-one years old at the time. His wife, June, was fifty-four. Bill had trouble adjusting to his new life circumstances, resulting in marital difficulties. However, with marriage counseling, Bill started coming around. Nevertheless, three years after the move, Bill still didn't feel quite settled, so the psychiatrist he had been seeing over the past year prescribed Prozac. He did not believe Bill to be suicidal or seriously depressed at that time.

After only two days on Prozac, Bill's condition deteriorated. He admitted himself to the hospital and stayed there for ten days. He was still on Prozac when they released him. The next day, when Bill and June failed to show up for a planned family outing, their son went to their home and found them. They were both dead, lying in a pool of blood. Eleven days after initiating Prozac therapy, Bill Forsyth had taken a serrated knife and stabbed his wife fifteen times. He then fixed the knife to a chair and impaled himself on it. Bill Forsyth, Jr. sued Eli Lilly for wrongful death.

During the trial, Eli Lilly's internal documentation revealed considerable awareness within the company about the risk of suicidal behavior. A letter sent to Eli Lilly in 1984 from the British Committee on Safety of Medicines read:

> During the treatment with [Prozac] 16 suicide attempts were made, two of these with success. As patients with a risk of suicide were excluded from the studies, it is probable that this high proportion can be attributed to an action of the preparation [medication].

In 1985, German authorities expressed concern about suicidal risks and required warnings of possible akathisia and suicide appear in the "Fluctin" (which is the German brand name for Prozac) labeling. Another document dated March 1985 suggested a rate of suicide for Prozac 5.6 times higher than for the older tricyclic antidepressants. It concluded "the benefits vs. risks considerations for fluoxetine [Prozac] currently [did] not fall clearly in favor of the benefits" (DeGrandpre). Sadly, none of these revelations would sway the jury to find Eli Lilly guilty of any wrongdoing. The plaintiffs lost their suit, and Eli Lilly once again walked away scot-free.

Additional Case Studies

One of the most comprehensive reviews I have read about the SSRIs and their dangers is Dr. Ann Blake Tracy's book, *Prozac: Panacea or Pandora?* She opens it with a profound, disturbing quote:

> I am alarmed at the monster that John Hopkins neuroscientist, Solomon Synder and I created when we discovered the simple binding assay for drug receptors 25 years ago (Tracy, 2001).

Why is it so chilling? Because this statement was made by Dr. Candace Pert, a research professor at Georgetown University Medical Center and past head of the brain chemistry department at the National Institute of Health (NIH). Dr. Pert was one of the discoverers of the SSRIs. She goes on to further state:

> Prozac and other antidepressant serotonin-receptor-active compounds may also cause cardiovascular problems in some susceptible people after long-term use, which has become common practice despite the lack of safety studies (Tracy, 2001).

Dr. Tracy is truly a heroine who has dedicated her profession and time to educating laymen and professionals alike on the dangers of the SSRIs. She has also served as an expert witness in some litigation. In her book, Dr. Tracy exposes a series of complications that have surfaced surrounding the use of these drugs and tells the moving anecdotal stories of victims who have been forever silenced. There is not room here to recount them all, but a couple of the following stories sound eerily familiar. So I have included them as additional evidence.

Fran Turner was a paramedic in Tacoma, Washington. Her life changed completely one night after she assisted a woman who had been stabbed and still had a knife embedded in her chest onto a hospital gurney. She ruptured a disc in her back. Fran was in her early thirties when the first operation was performed on her back. Nobody thought to ask her if she smoked or took birth control pills before administering anesthesia. That was Fran's first adverse drug reaction. The combination caused her to have a stroke. After several years of relearning to do things and living with continual back pain, Fran decided to see a psychiatrist. He prescribed Prozac. Fran had several grand mal seizures, the kind an epileptic might experience. She also listed a large number of side effects such as "total sleep deprivation, radical rise in depression, increase in muscle spasms (severe and prolonged) in L4–5 back, increase in spasms in left hip, increase in pain in both legs, decreased sensation in both feet, increase in (severe and prolonged) headaches, diarrhea, dehydration, total loss of appetite and alternating chills and sweating" (Tracy 240).

The list of drugs her doctor prescribed for her grew as she experienced more and more adverse side effects. Fran, still having some presence of mind, finally demanded she be taken off the drugs. Her psychiatrist refused. He insisted her family doctor should be the one to discontinue some of the drugs he was prescribing. Only days before she died, Fran, on her own, discontinued the Prozac, Halcion, Serax, Dilantin, Midrin, Lasix, and Vistaril she was taking. However, she continued taking the Darvocet, Soma, Lioresal, and Deseryl she had been prescribed.

Fran wrote the following note to her psychiatrist, just before she pulled a gun in his office and shot herself. It read:

> I was depressed so you fed me Prozac. I couldn't sleep so you gave me Halcion and Sinequan. Whenever I was pushed beyond my limits you ordered Serax. These drugs were your choice of treatment, not mine. If anybody is responsible for me staying on them for too long it's you, not me. Your course of treatment was to deal with the symptoms—not the underlying causes…The next time you order your favorite drugs for someone, think of me and be aware that patients need the counseling skills you've learned far more than the drugs your 'MD' allows you to cop-out with (Tracy 240–241).

Betty Broderick, a wealthy California woman, appeared on *The Oprah Winfrey Show* in the fall of 1992. Betty had broken into her ex-husband's bedroom in November 1989. She then shot and killed him and his new wife. Not one word was mentioned about the fact that Betty had been on Prozac at the time of the murders. Oprah's questions brought out all of the symptoms of Prozac adverse reactions reported by other Prozac survivors. Betty said all the classic things: She thought she was evil. She had intended to kill herself as well, but she did not have any bullets left in the gun. Betty also appeared to have no remorse, suggesting an inability to feel emotions or guilt. She displayed paranoid behavior, and she said she believed her husband was trying to ruin her. She even portrayed herself as the victim in the situation. Betty was described by others as being extremely narcissistic, that is, she lacked empathy and was unwilling to recognize the feelings and needs of others. All of these signs and symptoms have been exhibited by patients who were in trouble on Prozac (Tracy 239-240).

Emotional Blunting

One of the most prestigious preceptorships I attended was at the Bethesda Naval Academy in neurology. It was an awesome, hands-on experience and gave me further insight to the complex workings of the brain. As a neurology/cardiology specialist for Syntex Labs, I sold Ticlid (ticlopidine), a drug to prevent stroke. This added yet another dimension to my continued education and medical discovery of the human anatomy.

As I learned about the functioning of the various hemispheres and areas of the brain, I found out, not only memory, but emotion, affect (facial expression), and inhibition are all controlled by the limbic system in the frontal lobe of the brain. This is where we feel our experiences. This is also the area where our survival instincts originate. From an evolutionary standpoint, this part of the brain is designed to be our center for paranoia. The limbic system remains alert for environmental dangers and, if detected, mounts an emotional response (Whitaker 163). Furthermore, this is the part of the brain that tells us when to put the brakes on inappropriate behavior. This was relevant to me because, in addition to a loss of memory and cognitive function, I also experienced an emotional blunting, that is, somewhat of a mild chemical lobotomy, for several months after taking that chemical deluge of antidepressants.

Furthermore, I went through a period afterward in which I felt completely uninhibited and began behaving and dressing differently, in ways which were uncharacteristic for me. I spent money impulsively, sometimes recklessly. I was completely unconcerned about social or economic repercussions. However, once the chemical fog lifted, I was embarrassed and upset about my risky behavior and adventures. It was like waking up to an alternate reality in which I was acting out someone else's fantasies. All of a sudden, the observer self was back in touch, and the realization of my actions was painfully humiliating.

Experts in psychiatry have postulated this drug-induced emotional blunting was responsible for the systematic killings that took place at Columbine High School in 1999. One of the gunmen, Eric Harris, was reportedly taking Luvox, another new antidepressant. Eric's parents are now suing Solvay, the drug's manufacturer. Within hours of this news hitting the airwaves, the American Psychiatric Association refuted that theory and was quoted as saying:

> Despite a decade of research, there is little valid evidence to prove a causal relationship between the use of antidepressant medications and destructive behavior. On the other hand, there is ample evidence that undiagnosed and untreated mental illness exacts a heavy toll on those who suffer from these disorders as well as those around them (Healy, *Let Them Eat Prozac*, 175).

In June 2001, Andrea Yates, a Houston woman who drowned her five children in the bathtub, was suffering from severe postpartum depression. Andrea was taking a cocktail of psychoactive drugs, including Effexor, Zyban, Remeron, and Haldol. Effexor had been prescribed at one and a half times the maximum dose (Tracy, 2001). Her psychiatrist had just discontinued Andrea's Haldol two days before the murders. Andrea said she heard voices telling her to kill her kids. She did not appear to have any homicidal tendencies before this incident. Her husband and friends were stunned. When she appeared in court, Andrea seemingly had no remorse for her actions. She was sentenced to life in prison for the murder of her children at the age of thirty-six. Just recently, this case was reopened when it was discovered one of the expert psychiatrists had provided false testimony during the original trial.

This case represents a blatant failure by the system to help Andrea and protect the Yates children. Andrea had a history of hospitalizations for mental illness. In her unstable condition, the children should never have been left alone in this poor woman's care.

Another recent tragedy that occurred in late March 2005 involved a sixteen-year-old, Jeff Weise. After first killing his grandfather and his companion, Jeff went on a shooting rampage at Red Lake High School in Minnesota. No one knows what motivated Jeff to kill nine people before he shot himself. He didn't leave a note, but Jeff had suffered tremendous emotional pain and loss in his adolescence. His father had committed suicide four years before, and his mother is currently confined to a nursing home with a brain injury she suffered in an automobile accident. Weise had been admitted to a psychiatric ward in Thief River Falls in the summer of 2004 after he concerned friends with suicidal messages he had posted on the Internet. He was prescribed Prozac. Family members reported Jeff's dosage had recently been increased to 60 milligrams daily. "I can't help but think it was too much, that it must have set him off," an aunt told reporters ("Friend: School Shooter on Prozac").

Nearly every day, I read or hear about something else on the news related to violence or homicides that are committed by people taking antidepressants. Maybe it is like buying a new car in which you suddenly start noticing that model everywhere on the road. However, I cannot help but wonder how many people are making the connection. There is obvious emotional blunting that is being exhibited by these individuals and a pattern of crimes of violence committed by people under the influence of antidepressants. Someone should take a serious look into these statistics and establish this correlation as fact, once and for all.

It is particularly disconcerting to know that large numbers of our young people are currently returning from Iraq and being diagnosed with post-traumatic stress disorder (PTSD). These young men and women have already been desensitized to violence because of their exposure to war. Now, they will also be prescribed high-risk medications that, as an end result, could still make them (and/or their families) fatalities of the war, even though they managed to make it back home to American soil in one piece.

5

Confessions of an Rx Drug Pusher

"In the middle of the journey of our life,
I found myself in a dark wood,
for I had lost the right path."

—**Dante**

It is pretty safe to say an outside sales rep's life in the industry revolves around one major relationship, the relationship with his or her district manager. This individual can make or break a sales rep's motivation and self-esteem, and he or she controls a large percentage of that individual's income as well. Interestingly enough, as much as I hated structure, I excelled under some of the most hard-nosed leaders, who were mostly ex-military men, when others flailed under the pressure of their demands. Their high expectations appealed to the overachiever syndrome I had developed as a child. I literally worked myself to utter exhaustion at some points in my career, simply because I knew no less than that was expected from me!

I was fortunate to have started in the pharmaceutical industry under an old-school district manager who shot from the hip and never compromised his ethics. From the beginning, he made it clear to me that it was a grievous mistake to refer to any drug as safe. Nothing was further from the truth. Every drug, depending on the individual taking it, could prove to be deadly. He encouraged full disclosure and taught me to sell my products based on their merits instead of bad-mouthing my competition.

I respected this man immensely and a couple of other managers I worked under later in my career. However, when it came to this attitude, I found these managers to be the exception, unfortunately, not the rule. Most middle managers intended to attain their quotas at all costs, fearing humiliation and embarrassment at meetings in front of their sales reps and fellow managers. I remember a manager saying on more than one occasion, "If it were me, I'd do such and such (as he or she disclosed some "pearl" of impropriety)…but don't ever say I said so because I'll deny it!"

The ink was barely dry on my newly signed contract with McNeil Pharmaceutical, a subsidiary of Johnson & Johnson, before one of its popular NSAID drugs, Zomax (zomepirac), was recalled. The drug had enjoyed tremendous launch success, and reps had instructed office staff to take it for everything from menstrual cramps to headaches. The problem was that the drug was not indicated for acute pain. All of the clinical studies had been conducted on long-term use in arthritis patients. Reports of severe allergic reactions known as anaphylaxis began surfacing with the intermittent, or occasional, use of the drug in the general population. Several patients died as a result.

Sensitive to the recent Oraflex fiasco in which Eli Lilly covered up deaths due to liver failure from its NSAID in other countries and clinical trials, the FDA made a swift decision to pull Zomax from the market. My first assignment in the field was to retrieve all of my doctors' Zomax samples.

It should be noted that only ten percent of adverse reactions are true allergic reactions. These are reactions in which the body mounts an attack against the drug as though it was a foreign invader. When this happens, anaphylactic shock occurs. Most drug reactions are attributable to overdoses or poisonings caused by an interaction between two or more substances (Fried 27).

Close on the heels of that recall, I was required to pick up all of the over-the-counter Tylenol in my territory because of the Chicago Tylenol poisonings. (McNeil Pharmaceutical and McNeil Consumer Products are both Johnson & Johnson companies.) This time, McNeil had voluntarily issued the massive recall. As a result, tamper-resistant packaging became mandatory for all over-the-counter products.

However, that was not to be the end of my recall experience with McNeil. The next product to be recalled would hit much closer to home. It was another NSAID called Suprol (suprofen). This was my first new drug launch. I remember the pride and exuberance I felt at the national launch meeting in which loudspeakers pumped out motivating theme music and medical researchers and marketing managers gave exciting, emotional speeches. I soaked in every word with anticipation and awe. I believed this drug was really going to help people!

During the breaks, scientists and corporate executives chatted amiably with reps while feasting on an elaborate array of snacks and beverages. Sumptuous gourmet meals and nightly entertainment further catered to the already inflated egos of the sales force. Open bars accompanied every event. T-shirts and ball caps emblazoned with the Suprol logo were distributed, along with sports bags that would transport all the rep's acquired goodies back home.

Pumped full of enthusiasm and focused on the key opinion leaders in my community, I returned to my territory. I bombarded them with studies and marketing materials in an effort to find support for my new drug. Marketing direction was very specific. Doctors in each territory had been profiled prior to the launch, and I was well-informed as to who the Early Adopters and High-Volume Prescribers (HVPs) of NSAIDs were. I was also aware of marketing's last-ditch effort directive to ask a reluctant prescriber to give me just one new start patient, even if it was his or her most difficult patient that had failed other therapies. The rationale was, if a doctor had success in one of his or her most difficult patients, he or she would be more inclined to write prescriptions for additional patients.

One of my doctors who practiced in a small, coastal town wrote large numbers of anti-inflammatory drugs for his predominantly geriatric population. He was an older doc himself, very nice, but set in his ways. He had been profiled as a Late Adopter/Skeptic. After a lengthy debate about the benefits of my new product, he shared his philosophy with me, which was not to prescribe a new drug until it had been on the market for a full year. This way, he could avoid the initial unknown complications that invariably surfaced with each new product. In other words, he preferred a "better safe than sorry" approach.

Still, I persisted in my enthusiasm and, as I had been instructed, asked for that "most difficult patient." I didn't leave until the doctor had committed to try the drug on at least one patient. He did finally commit, or, to use sales jargon, I closed him. I left triumphant…or so I thought.

I continued drumming up support for Suprol and had just gotten it added to my major teaching hospital's formulary when I got the bad news. An emergency teleconference was called, and the company announced a "Dear Doctor" letter would be sent to all physicians that day addressing "new complications" associated with Suprol, primarily flank pain. Nearly twenty-five percent of the patients affected had required hospitalization. Flank pain is a very serious side effect because it indicates the possibility of kidney damage.

Little did I know at the time, one of the doctors who had reported an adverse event, which eventually resulted in death due to dialysis complications, was in my territory. I was later contacted and instructed by management to have my doctor complete an Adverse Drug Reaction (ADR) report. Much to my surprise, the doctor referenced in my instructions was the Late Adopter/Skeptic, who had promised me his "most difficult patient" against his better judgment. Even more startling would be the discovery that the patient had been his very own mother. Of course, I didn't find that out until I visited him to do the ADR. (By the way, the ADR was a daunting ream of paperwork that appeared to be designed to discourage busy doctors from reporting.) I will never forget the betrayed look on his face or his terse remark to me that "the company's marketing strategy had obviously been more thoroughly tested than our drug!" I was devastated and riddled with guilt. I didn't call on his office again for nearly six months. I didn't have the nerve!

Suprol was eventually recalled in 1987 after it had first been banned in Europe. I found myself backpedaling in offices, once again embarrassed as I picked up samples. Reps were instructed to take a proactive stance with providers by pointing out the swift, decisive action taken by the company to remove the product once the adverse events surfaced. What reps were not told was that Public Citizen, Ralph Nader's consumer activist organization, had actually sued the FDA in order to protect consumers and have Suprol pulled from the market.

So, I was somewhat surprised later on to discover that not all of my pharmaceutical cohorts in the marketing and sales departments subscribed to the Hippocratic Oath: "First, do no harm." Marketing strategies were designed to do one thing: maximize profits. If information could have a negative impact on the bottom line, reps were instructed to downplay it. The opposite was true of even the most ridiculous perceived benefit. Patent extensions were sought for minute enhancements, and tons of marketing hoopla would tout the "new and improved" products.

A good example would be the relaunch of Prozac under the new name of Sarafem. The drugs are exactly the same chemical, but, because the patent on Prozac was about to expire, it allowed Eli Lilly to capture a market where its new product was exclusively protected by patent. A new disease state emerged that was essentially created for marketing purposes, premenstrual dysphoric disorder (PMDD). Before the Sarafem launch, PMDD did not exist in any diagnostic textbooks.

Prescription for Sales Success

I wouldn't want to misrepresent the entire pharmaceutical profession. Many of the closest friendships I formed over the years were with colleagues in this industry. They were intelligent, hard-working, dedicated citizens who wanted to do something that made a contribution while providing an above-average income for their families. At one time, I believed, as do most pharmaceutical reps, what I was doing helped people. Like many of them, I wanted to be as informed and well-educated as possible in my profession. I spent numerous hours studying and reading, and I subscribed to several prestigious journals to stay abreast of current literature. However, this was later in my career when my audience of specialists was a little more challenging than the average family practitioner. The specialists were well-read doctors, and they asked lots of critically intelligent questions. So, in anticipation of their objections, I asked lots of questions and attempted to have a better grasp of my customers' needs.

I recall an early encounter with a young, marketing executive in the now-defunct Syntex Laboratories. We were at a company-wide sales meeting. Nearly 1,000 reps from around the country were in attendance. He was discussing the dosing recommendations for an NSAID that was a counterpart to the then the number one seller for arthritis, Naprosyn (naproxen). The drug's name was Anaprox DS (naproxen sodium). It is currently sold over-the-counter in less than half the prescription strength as Aleve.

Anaprox is the same chemical compound as Naprosyn. The only difference is the sodium added to improve absorption time. Therefore, Anaprox is promoted for acute, short-term pain. The drug has a twelve-hour half-life. That means it takes at least twelve hours following administration for the body to eliminate fifty percent of the drug. After that, blood levels of the drug fall below their therapeutic range. A drug with a twelve-hour half-life would require a b.i.d., or twice daily, dosing regimen in order to sustain blood levels and maximize therapeutic efficacy. The Anaprox dosage recommendation, however, was t.i.d., or three times daily. This prompted me to ask the product manager, "Why?"

Initially, he disregarded my question and responded, "Because we can. We sell more pills that way." He then moved on; however, I persisted and raised my hand again. To his annoyance, I asked, "Doesn't that unnecessarily increase the possibility of GI [gastrointestinal] complications such as bleeding and ulceration?" His next remark would haunt me for the remainder of my career, "Well, of course it does," he said chuckling, "but, luckily for those patients, we have a new H2-blocker in the pipeline!" The crowd erupted in laughter, and I made a mental note to ask one of my older colleagues what exactly an H2-blocker was.

During the next coffee break, I discovered H2-blockers (H2-antagonists) were designed to treat stomach ulcerations. The company, indeed, had one in licensing negotiations. Whether this statement was jocular in nature or not, it revealed an underlying attitude that was pervasive in the industry and would surface time and again in my experience. Patients were regarded as consumers and, as such, were a dispensable human commodity.

Ironically enough, I would be the victim of my own wares with this product. Because of my indiscriminate use of Anaprox samples for headaches and back pain, I had a serious GI bleed in 1990. Included in the irony was the fact it happened to me during a training program while I was at the Syntex corporate offices in Palo Alto. I realize now it was real-life training for me.

During my research for this book, I discovered more than 16,000 patients die annually from the use of prescription and over-the-counter NSAIDs. I also learned more than 100,000 hospital admissions yearly could be attributed to GI bleeding from NSAIDs alone (Strand 173). Although I knew about the risk of GI bleeding and ulceration, the gravity of these statistics was never brought to my attention by any of the companies for which I sold NSAIDs.

A Loss of Innocence: Ida Smith's Story

At the beginning of my career, I was a field rep in Corpus Christi, Texas. I sold a variety of medications, including Haldol (haloperidol) for schizophrenia and senile dementia. My territory, with the exception of Corpus Christi, was primarily rural. It included several small towns in the outlying countryside. The demographics of the area were largely Hispanics and the elderly who came south for the winter months.

It was the end of the third quarter, and I was behind in my sales quota for Haldol. That meant forfeiting a significant amount of money from the bonus pool if I didn't make quota. My territory was at somewhat of a disadvantage because I didn't have the large number of psychiatrists the reps in other metropolitan areas such as Dallas, Houston, and Austin had. It occurred to me that the most common drawback/objection I received from the general practitioners I called on with this product was patient compliance. (Patients would frequently discontinue the medication because of its side effects.) So, I determined the best way to build my Haldol business would be to campaign for the institutionalized patient. These patients were not only encouraged to take the medication; they were actually given the drug. This completely eliminated the compliance issue.

I set about scheduling training in-services in the local nursing homes and mental health and mental retardation (MHMR) facilities. I increased my call frequency on physicians whom I knew to have nursing home relationships and directorship responsibilities. I littered these offices and institutions with every type of marketing tool known to man. You could not look anywhere in my territory that there wasn't a clock, coffee mug, calendar, candy dish, scratch pad, or pen displaying the Haldol name.

During my so-called "Haldol Blitz," I made weekly visits to my nursing homes. The nursing staff was very supportive and appreciated being the recipients of all the goodies and attention that was rarely placed on them. (Reps notoriously do not like to call on nursing homes or abortion clinics.) They began to eagerly recommend to doctors that patients be placed on Haldol and actually kept track of patients who were put on the drug to report to me on subsequent visits. I rewarded these facilities and staffs with catered-in lunches and gift certificates to local restaurants.

In my routine visits to one particular nursing home, I met Mrs. Ida Smith. (I have changed her name to protect her privacy.) Mrs. Smith was a petite, fragile-looking woman in her late eighties. Her snow-white hair was always neatly coiffed. She also wore a bright red lipstick that contrasted starkly with her delicate, pale complexion. Ida was a whirlwind of activity in her motorized wheelchair. She was frequently seen motoring from room to room, checking on and visiting with other residents. It was apparent the nursing staff was put out with Mrs. Smith's meddling. Ida often complained to staff about patients who were not properly being cared for. She was the self-appointed hall monitor and was not afraid to let people know she was watching. I got a kick out of observing the nurses' reactions when Mrs. Smith would demand someone change a bedpan or IV bag that had been left unattended. She could definitely hold her own in a debate.

Mrs. Smith became a bright spot in my visits to an otherwise gloomy, depressing facility that reeked with the stench of urine and disinfectant. However, I called on the home one day, and Mrs. Smith was nowhere to be seen. Before departing, I questioned the head nurse about her. "Oh, Mrs. Smith, she's had a bad patch lately," she said. "Her friend in 17B died, and it really upset her. She hadn't been sleeping well and seemed a little disoriented, so we recommended her doctor put her on Haldol. She's doing a lot better now…sleeping through the night…not combative and quarrelsome like she used to be." She concluded, smiling. (It was obvious she thought she was making brownie points with me.)

As I rounded the corner to the front door, I saw an attendant pushing Mrs. Smith in her wheelchair into her room. Her head was hung, and she was drooling on her pretty, pink gown. Mrs. Smith looked like a *zombie*. She was in complete disarray. Her hair was uncombed, and her signature red lipstick was missing. I felt a pang in the pit of my stomach. Had I been responsible for this turn of events? Surely, Mrs. Smith was not the patient-type for whom I had promoted Haldol. Or was she?

I exceeded my quota in all four of my products that sales quarter. Shortly thereafter, I was promoted to a hospital rep's position in Houston for the Baylor College of Medicine. I would never see Mrs. Smith again. However, my last memory of her would stay fresh in my mind and on my conscience for many years to come.

Selling Out for Sales

For the majority of my career, I sold what I considered, at the time, to be fairly innocuous drugs, even though, as I said previously, I sold several NSAIDs, which are known to kill thousands of people annually and hospitalize tens of thousands more. Over the course of the years, my knowledge base would expand with each new category of drug I sold as I learned about the disease states and the body systems affected by each drug. The flip side of this was that, if I hadn't sold a particular drug or competed with that category with one of my products, I was as ignorant as the next guy about what it did, how it worked, what risks were associated with its use, and so forth.

One of the advantages I enjoyed while working with a number of key manufacturers was having exceptional training programs. Had I stayed with one company, I would not have had the diversity of product knowledge and variety of sales training I ultimately received. Looking back, I would realize the buyouts, downsizings, layoffs, and ultimate challenges that had forced me to change employment several times had given me a phenomenal array of medical education. In the span of fifteen years, I had promoted NSAIDs, narcotic analgesics, antibiotics, asthma drugs, muscle relaxants, antihypertensive agents, lipid-lowering statins, antifungal preparations, birth control pills, diabetes drugs, hormone replacement therapy, stroke treatments, and, of course, neuroleptic drugs. I had worked my way up the corporate ladder, starting with my first promotion from a territory rep to a hospital rep after only eighteen months with McNeil. Then, with Syntex, I was promoted to an ob-gyn specialist. Before being severed, I worked as a cardiology and neurology specialist. I was hired as a cardiology and diabetes specialist with Bristol-Myers Squibb. In nine months, I received the Pinnacle Award, which was given to the top three percent of its sales force. At the end of my career, as an independent contractor, I became an overdressed sample delivery girl. Basically, I was paid per signature. Well, actually, I was paid per call, but I needed to get a doctor's signature in order to prove I had been there.

Out of all of the drugs I had sold over the years in various specialties, the only drug that ever really challenged my moral ethics was Haldol, particularly Haldol decanoate. This was the "Big Daddy" of all neuroleptics. It made me cringe while learning about this newest form of Haldol during the launch meeting when I envisioned the possible torture in store for some patients. As I indicated earlier, patient non-compliance was a fairly common drawback with Haldol treatment. The side effects of neuroleptic drugs can be absolutely unbearable.

As a hospital rep, I would frequently see institutionalized patients pacing frantically back and forth in waiting rooms, hallways, and outside in foyers. Some would literally wear the soles off of their house shoes. Others would fall sound asleep prostrate on the ground, wherever they were when the drug's sedative effects hit. Patients frequently drooled, sat staring into space, experienced facial grimacing, or continually made pill-rolling motions between their thumbs and forefingers. I soon realized many of the bizarre behaviors and movements I had previously identified with schizophrenia and other mental illness were entirely the fault of the medications the patients were taking. They were not a manifestation of these disorders.

Once, I encountered a twelve-year-old boy in the emergency room who had taken his grandmother's medication. His eyes had rolled into the back of his head and locked there. This is known as an oculogyric crisis. However, where my heart really went out was to the poor, little elderly patients in the Veterans Administration (VA) hospital, the nursing homes, and the psychiatric wards. They seemed to suffer the most on Haldol. I heard constant reports about excessive dry mouth, blurry vision, painful constipation, and urinary retention. (Nurses even complained about fecal impacts associated with chronic neuroleptic use.) These side effects are known as anticholinergic effects, and my training had actually consisted of a little rhyme to assist me in learning them. It went, "Patients on Haldol can't see, can't spit, can't pee, and can't shit."

Reps were instructed to minimize these side effects by encouraging the doctor to simply administer an anticholinergic drug simultaneously with Haldol. Still, the most dreaded side effect by patients and doctors alike remained akathisia. A patient with agitated akathisia could not only be self-injurious, but was also a danger to other patients and staff.

These observations lead me to question the medical prudence and moral ethics behind giving a long-acting, irreversible neuroleptic like Haldol decanoate, especially because Haldol was documented to have a huge potential to cause negative side effects. Once this drug was on board and a patient reacted to it, there was absolutely nothing doctors could do except give additional drugs to manage the side effects while the patient rode out the three weeks the injection was intended to last. Of course, three weeks was only the half-life of the drug. There would be remaining drug residual for some time after that.

The company's position was that the untreated schizophrenic patient is a threat to society and himself. Traditional oral medications could not ensure patient compliance in the absence of an institutional setting. With larger numbers of mental health patients being forced into outpatient settings such as

MHMR facilities, there seemed to be a real, perceived need for this extended-release form of Haldol. Hence, the product managers argued the benefits outweighed the risks, particularly when you considered one of the benefits was that Haldol decanoate would enjoy an exclusive patent whereas the old haloperidol was available generically and sold at a significant cost reduction. Not only did Haldol decanoate ensure patient compliance, it ensured corporate longevity as well. Back then, at an average wholesale cost of $165 per injection, Haldol decanoate was a much more profitable dosage form than the tablet counterpart that sold for pennies on the dollar. The marketing strategy revealed at launch was to acquire the stabilized patient, emphasizing the reduced chance of relapse and overall reduced drug exposure. (Why? Were they admitting drug exposure was harmful to the patient?) That meant getting the long-term refill business. Never mind that the long-acting neuroleptics were already known to cause even worse side effects than their shorter-acting versions. For the company, this was considered a small price to pay for the trade-off.

Being the ambitious, determined person I was, I set out to convert as much of my Haldol tablet business to Haldol decanoate business as I could. In spite of my reservations, I justified the activity because I figured it wasn't my place to question the treatment choices made by a patient's doctor. That's not what I was paid to do. I was only there to provide the information to help him or her make the best choices, right? So true! But, even then, only two years into the game, I was already beginning to question: The best choices for whom?

6

Anxiolytics: Prescription for Addiction

"Addiction [is] a preoccupation and compulsive use of an experience or substance despite the recurrence of adverse consequences...some people may have a biological or genetic predisposition to addiction."

—The ASAP Dictionary of Anxiety and Panic Disorders

My first basic sales training class with McNeil found me roommates with a former Upjohn rep. We got along well, and her previous experience was a comfort to a novice rep like me. Under the pressure of the long hours and lack of sleep, I started getting anxious. After all, I wasn't able to take pot on my business trips, my usual way of winding down for the evening in order to relax and sleep. My roommate, on the other hand, had the perfect solution. Upjohn had a new anxiolytic called Xanax (alprazolam). It was being touted as the nonaddicting Valium. They were also marketing a new sleep aid in the same drug category called Halcion (triazolam). (The industry had coined the term anxiolytic because of the negative publicity benzodiazepines were receiving about their addiction potential.) My roommate had samples of both and offered me some.

I remembered my mother giving me her Valium (diazepam) once before a beauty pageant I was in. I was fourteen. It felt wonderful. The total calm and the jitteriness that often consumed me were completely relieved as I confidently glided across stage. I loved it! I popped the Xanax without a second thought. Sure enough, I loved it too! As for the Halcion, I would sleep the sleep of the dead that night. I don't think I have ever slept that well since. I would refrain from taking Halcion too much after overhearing a conversation between two residents that had pulled long shifts the day and night before. One would confide to the other that he had found notes in one of the patient's charts that he had written the previous night, but he had no memory of having been called back to the hospital. The other resident had kind of laughed and shrugged it off, but I could tell the doctor involved was really disturbed by his memory malfunction. I decided to limit my Halcion use to rare occasions as needed.

These drugs would be my mainstay, off and on, for the next ten years. Somehow, I felt less guilty and more dignified about using these drugs over marijuana. They were the perfect solution for me. They were not illegal. I didn't have to worry about the random drug testing I underwent in the industry. They didn't make me have glassy, red eyes. There was no stigma attached to taking them, and they didn't impair my mental functioning (or so I thought) the way marijuana did. I could take these things all day long if needed whereas I could only smoke pot at the end of the evening or after I had completed my day's work.

One time, my dentist, my dermatologist, my family practitioner, and my ob-gyn all prescribed Xanax for various things. My dentist gave me a script before a dental procedure he thought might cause anxiety. My dermatologist did the same before sclera therapy, a procedure to repair spider veins. My ob-gyn wrote one for PMS symptoms, and my family practitioner prescribed it for sleep disturbance. I remember I didn't even fill all of the scripts because I had so much Xanax.

Upjohn heavily promoted both Halcion and Xanax for years. Samples of Xanax would literally fall off of shelves because they were so crammed into sample closets! However, that soon changed as other reps caught wind of the drugs' wonders and became addicted. Samples began falling into open detail bags instead of patient's hands, making them more and more difficult to find. Some doctors would readily give samples to reps for anything we complained about, including work stressors, back pain, sleep problems, and so forth. Of course, with time, it would be discovered short-acting benzodiazepines are even more addicting than long-acting ones like Valium.

Additionally, controversy that surfaced surrounding Halcion and drug-induced psychosis resulted in the drug being banned in the United Kingdom in 1993. Thirteen other countries followed this action. Partially, this occurred for reasons that emerged in the 1988 trial of Ilo Grundberg, a fifty-seven-year-old Utah woman who killed her elderly mother by shooting her eight times in the head. Grundberg was judged to have been "involuntarily intoxicated" by Halcion, and Upjohn settled out of court in 1991. However, documentation uncovered in the discovery process of the trial disclosed a clinical study submitted for Halcion's approval that had "underreported the number of patients who had paranoid reactions to the drug and overstated the number who had similar reactions to a placebo." In spite of the paperwork discrepancies, the FDA still considered Halcion safe and effective following its investigation (Fried 239).

Believe it or not, I still didn't know I was *addicted* to Xanax for several years. When I discovered I was pregnant in 1988 with my son, out of concern for the fetus, I stopped taking it cold turkey. Boy, that would turn out to be a mistake!

The panic attacks started almost immediately. I had been on Xanax for nearly three years. I thought I was going to die! My heart raced, and my hands shook. I thought I would suffocate. I was short of breath and dizzy. I had a total loss of spatial perception. I had no idea what was happening! I started getting seriously anxious and mildly depressed. I couldn't sleep. I was under a tremendous amount of pressure at work at the time, in addition to the pregnancy, so I attributed it to that. I sought out a psychologist to talk to. She diagnosed me with an adjustment disorder. With her assistance, I managed to get through the next several weeks of withdrawal hell. Talk about morning sickness! I would vomit, and I was nauseous from daylight to dark that first three months. In fact, the doctors were concerned I was losing, not gaining, weight with the pregnancy. Nobody had even thought to consider I might be experiencing drug withdrawal, even though, at some point, I had informed all of my caretakers I had been taking Xanax. Because these drug-induced symptoms resembled the same ones associated with the problems for which I had been prescribed Xanax, I remained clueless as well. I would discover much later that any psychiatric symptom or disorder can also be *caused* by the drugs used to treat them (Breggin and Cohen 50).

It should be noted that dependence on anxiolytics/benzodiazepines can develop rapidly, often within days or weeks. All long-term users are addicted. Benzodiazepine withdrawals are considered far worse and last much longer than those associated with alcohol or barbiturates. They can sometimes last weeks or months, depending on the length of time the drug has been used. Other commonly prescribed benzodiazepines include Serax (oxazepam), Klonopin (clonazepam), Ativan (lorazepam), Dalmane (flurazepam), Restoril (temazepam), Tranxene (clorazepate), ProSom (estazolam), Librium (chlordiazepoxide), and Versed (midazolam) (Kotulak).

Addiction and Mental Illness

Mental illness seems to occur more frequently in substance users. Once again, it is the age-old "chicken or the egg" dilemma. Did the drugs cause the condition, or did the condition predispose the individual to drug use? The fact is that it can be extremely difficult to discern which came first. However, many substance abusers describe being driven to drug or alcohol use in order to manage their mood swings or deal with feelings of inadequacy. This process of self-medicating contributes to substance abuse and addiction in many people with mood disorders.

Addiction is not a moral weakness of character or lack of self-control. If you have a brain, you have the potential to become an addict. Addiction, as we have seen, is also not limited to illicit drugs. Many of the prescription psychoactive drugs and hypnotic pain killers are highly addicting. Our drug rehabilitation and psychiatric treatment facilities can attest to that. It is no secret in the medical community that drug addiction among professionals is highest among their own, including doctors, nurses, drug reps, and pharmacists, who all have easy access to controlled prescription medications (Kuhn et al 254–255).

Becoming a Mother in the Eye of a Hurricane

I was about eight-and-a-half months pregnant when my husband's daughters from his first marriage were taken from his first wife in Wisconsin. She had a cocaine addiction and was neglecting her children. Her two sons by her second husband had already been sent to live with their father. The youngest daughter, Connie, came to live with us in Corpus Christi while the older daughter, Tina, went to live with my husband's parents near Milwaukee.

It was a difficult transition for Connie at the age of twelve. Not only was she a long distance from her home in Wisconsin, but it was the first time she had been separated from her sister, Tina, who was very close to her in age. Connie was also very attached to her younger brothers. As it were, she had been their caretaker, and now they were also gone. It was heartbreaking when she arrived with all of her worldly belongings in one small brown box. Most of it, odds and ends of clothing and junk jewelry, was not even worth keeping. I bought her a new ward-robe and got her hair cut stylishly. I set about trying to make her over. Poor thing, now that I look back, I had no idea how that must have made her feel. I meant well, and the little girl in me so wanted her acceptance. However, I am pretty sure she interpreted it as though she was not good enough for me the way she was.

Connie was a good little helper. I could tell she had been given responsibility for her siblings and housework because she assisted with little complaint. She understandably felt a loyalty toward her mother, even though I had not been party to the separation between Connie's parents. She resented my relationship with her father, partly because I think she felt abandoned by him. Rod had joined the navy to support the children shortly after the divorce. They were very young, only four and five years old, when he was stationed in Hawaii. The girls had endured unspeakable neglect and abuse when they were left in their mother's sole custody. My husband and I were shocked at the information Connie shared with us. He really had not known the extent of her mother's dysfunction and addiction since their divorce. So, it was also understandable that Connie had grown a thick skin at an early age to protect herself. All of my attempts to break through to her were thwarted.

Nevertheless, I enjoyed having Connie around and getting a head start on parenting, although it would be quite different trying to mentor a twelve-year-old girl that resented me from caring for a totally dependent infant boy that was soon to arrive. It was a blessing to have Connie as a part of our family at that time. I hope she will someday see it that way. She was there for the birth of her half-brother, but, unfortunately, she was also there for my postpartum depression.

I guess everything in my life was intended to be high drama because I didn't even manage to have my son under normal circumstances. On September 11, 1988, (notice the poor kid's birthday) when our son, Austin, entered the world, Corpus Christi was being evacuated in anticipation of the arrival of Hurricane Gilbert. It was predicted we would be in the eye of the storm any day. I was in the hospital hooked up to an intravenous Pitocin-drip in an attempt to induce labor. Because I had gestational diabetes, the doctor was concerned. I was overdue, and the baby might get too large, further complicating the delivery.

Several hours later, eighteen to be exact, they disconnected the IV and told me to go home. It was obvious the baby was not coming. I had not even dilated one centimeter after eighteen hours of killer contractions produced by the Pitocin. Maybe the drop in barometric pressure would induce labor. I was told to go home and wait.

We had no sooner gotten home before, lo and behold, my water broke. So, it was back to the hospital for labor and delivery. The only problem was that I still wasn't dilating. The pain was so excruciating. I guess I was controlling it. Finally, the doctor on call arrived and sent for the anesthesiologist.

I remember curling up into a ball as I waited in anticipation, attempting not to move while the spinal block was started. Sweet relief! I was so relieved that I started to dilate instantly. One...two...three...four centimeters...

The doctor was alarmed. "Somebody put an IV in her!" he barked. "This baby's coming!"

The nurses scrambled to get the IV in, but, because I was so dehydrated, they had to make several attempts until they finally settled for a vein in the top of my hand. The coaches were telling me to push—push with all my might! The baby was just starting to crown.

Suddenly, the doctor looked startled as he watched the monitor of the baby's heartbeat.

"Something's happening...something's wrong...I can feel it," I thought.

"The baby's in distress," he said. "We can't wait...Forceps!"

I thought I would faint. Then, all at once, the baby was out. His umbilical cord was wrapped around his neck, and the doctor quickly untied it. I saw the medical personnel shoving my husband out the door into the foyer as he objected. The baby was immediately swept away by the nurses and was not placed on my stomach as I had seen in my prenatal films. That was when my ears started to fill with fluid, as though I was being submerged under water. I tried verbalizing this to the doctor.

"Damn it, Gwen, stay with me!" he demanded. "We're losing her," I heard him say to the anesthesiologist as his voice faded with everything else and the room went black.

I didn't see any tunnels or lights, nor did I have any deceased relatives come to greet me. However, at that instant, I was consumed with an utter feeling of peace I have only had once since. That would be the night I talked with God. I experienced the dissolution of my individual boundaries and felt a complete oneness with everything around me. I no longer felt separated physically from anyone or anything in the room. I had no fear and no apprehension. It was just a wonderful, blissful feeling of peace. I would never again be afraid to die.

When I came to, all of these ashen-white faces were hovering above me with frightened, concerned looks on them. Apparently, I had lost a considerable amount of blood. My uterus had been seriously torn by the forceps. I was also having an allergic reaction to the Duramorph (morphine sulfate), the anesthesia in my spinal block.

The next several hours would be touch-and-go for me. I was hooked up to a monitor that would sound an alarm to staff when I stopped breathing. And I did stop breathing frequently. I broke out in an itchy rash all over my body. Benadryl was added to my IV to control the itching and swelling. Breast-feeding was out of the question because I was too weak to even sit up for long periods of time. So, I was given Parlodel, a drug to dry up my breast milk. (This was an "off-label" indication that eventually got the drug recalled for causing strokes in healthy postpartum women.) It would be ten hours before I was allowed to see or hold my baby. All that was a cakewalk compared to the postpartum depression that would follow later.

(Doctors can prescribe any drug to any patient for any condition he or she deems appropriate. This is legal even though the drug may only be officially approved for specific indications for which it has been tested. Drug companies heavily promote "off-label" and sometimes untested uses of drugs. It is another area in which drug reps often utilize key opinion leaders in order to establish a drug's off-label indications.)

When my son was four days old, I was discharged from the hospital. We went to Austin (the city) to stay with friends and escape Hurricane Gilbert and the spin-off of tornadoes that would surely follow the hurricane. I was extremely weak and developed a uterine infection to further complicate my condition. The usual four-hour trip between Corpus Christi and Austin had been much longer, tedious, and crowded, as evacuees fled from the coast to inland cities. Hurricane Gilbert eventually hit land in Brownsville, further south of Corpus. So, the trek home was uneventful. Fortunately, our apartment had not sustained any damage.

My recovery from the complications during labor and delivery was slow. Although I was basically elated to be alive and have a healthy baby, an emotional storm was brewing internally that I couldn't put a finger on. Yes, there were stressors resulting from Connie and the baby, but something else was happening. I couldn't control my ruminating thoughts of sad, painful, disturbing memories. I was consumed by overwhelming despair and "gloom and doom" feelings. It took all of my energy and effort just to get out of bed, much less care for my infant son and twelve-year-old stepdaughter. I also felt irritable and teary-eyed, and would explode into uncontrollable sobbing without provocation. Now I really thought I was losing it! Moreover, I identified this behavior with my mother and her mother, and worried incessantly about my newborn baby.

"You're *crazy*, just like your mother," echoed the familiar phrase repeatedly in my head. I fought so hard just to act normal!

Connie was unable to adjust to her new environment, and she was lonely for her siblings. She began to act out and eventually returned to Wisconsin. Our relationship with Connie became more and more distant as the years passed. As an adult, she changed her name and moved. We lost total contact with her. Tina would keep in touch sporadically over the years.

Both of my husband's daughters struggled with emotional problems in their adolescence and adult lives. Tina also had her own bout with alcohol and drug abuse, and she was forced to spend several months in a juvenile rehabilitation/ detention center. We would bear an immense sense of guilt and responsibility. At the time, I was a wounded young woman myself. It is painful to admit, but, at that point, I didn't think it was my responsibility to rescue Rod's children. We certainly didn't do enough, but could we have spared them from some of their more painful childhood lessons? I'm not sure. In hindsight, my heart would later question, "What if we had taken both of them?" Once again, there are always lots of "what ifs" to be reflected on down the road. Always in hindsight, the truth is revealed and as it is often quoted, "The truth hurts."

7

Another One Flew Over the Cuckoo's Nest: Geraldine's Story

"I must be crazy to be in a loony bin like this."

—**McMurphy,** *One Flew Over the Cuckoo's Nest* **(1975)**

I have long since determined the only thing that probably saved my sanity and/or my life was my ability to stay out of the psychiatric hospital. Believe me, I fought like hell to do that! All of my doctors encouraged me to be institutionalized in 1992. Of course, it was for my own safety. The impressions of psychiatric facilities that haunted me were the result of my exposure to them in my experience selling Haldol with McNeil, as much as they were disturbing remnants of my childhood memories.

The calls always came in the middle of the night. My grandmother had attempted suicide or had gone off the deep end again and required hospitalization. Because we were a working-class family, that meant admission to the state hospital. It was a dreary, depressing compound of buildings. The cold, austere feeling of the environment alone terrified me as a child, not to mention the moaning, screams, and other bizarre behaviors I had witnessed from the patients when visiting.

Because we lived in Indiana and Mamaw lived in Ohio, it was several hours drive before we would get to Toledo. We usually went straight to the hospital. Depending on the severity of the breakdown, I was often encouraged to visit. Sometimes my grandmother would be in a stupor—uncommunicative and expressionless—as she sat staring into the distance. Other times, she would be babbling incoherent, nonsensical conversation with anyone who would listen. It not only scared me, but it broke my heart to see my grandmother that way.

Mamaw was an intelligent, warm, humorous human being when she wasn't sick. She loved to play cards and had taught me the game of canasta when my hands were barely big enough to hold the spread of cards. More and more as the years passed, I sensed her slipping away. The person she had been no longer existed. What remained was a brain-damaged, confused, and pathetic shell of a person who spent the majority of her time smoking cigarettes, smacking her lips, and staring off into space. It was extremely sad.

My relationship with Mamaw had been forever marred by a childhood wounding I could not forgive. Even though I knew she was ill, I would hold her morally responsible for the insane way she treated me during the Christmas of 1971.

My grandfather, Junie, was a big, jovial man who smelled like exotic pipe tobacco and cheap men's cologne. As a little girl, I adored him and would slip my soft, little hands into his large, calloused palms when we walked together or climb onto his lap any chance I got. I heard stories about his philandering when he was young, but that never curbed my enthusiasm about Papaw. We didn't see each other often, and I never knew anything except kindness and humor from him.

That Christmas, I was invited to travel in my grandparents' motor home to Florida and vacation over the holiday. The first part of the trip was mostly uneventful. Mamaw and I played cards while chatting nonstop as Papaw drove the RV. I remember her raucous laughter that frequently erupted into hacking, coughing spells caused by a chronic bronchitis.

We stopped in Atlanta at a shopping mall to buy Christmas presents. Mamaw bought me a really cool pair of red, stretch, bell-bottom pants and a matching, flowered, button-down blouse that would be my favorite outfit that year. The weather in Florida was balmy and warm when we arrived at our campsite. Life was good, at least for a little while.

My memory of the details from here on gets sketchy except for the most traumatic highlights. Only a couple of days after we arrived in Florida, Mamaw began behaving oddly. She seemed agitated and argumentative. She had difficulty sleeping and would keep Papaw up all night talking. She would then bustle about to-and-fro as she engaged in meaningless activity the entire next day.

Papaw began worrying Mamaw either wasn't taking her drugs or she wasn't doing well on the new drugs she had been given most recently. He told me we needed to think about heading home early. By the time we packed our things and embarked on our long road trip back to Ohio, Mamaw was completely manic psychotic.

She accused me of sexual improprieties with Papaw. I was only twelve. I was mortified at the very suggestion and deeply wounded by her accompanying verbal attack. I remember the cynical tone in her voice as she hurled her vicious accusations, "I know he wants to screw you!" she hissed. "…you let him, too, didn't you? You little whore!"

I wanted to die! I could not process what was happening to me. This Dr. Jekyll and Mr. Hyde transformation had taken place in only a matter of days! How could she treat me this way? What had I done to deserve this?

Mamaw wouldn't allow me to eat or sleep at all. When it was dark out, she would hold a flashlight in my eyes as we rolled seemingly endless hours through the night toward home. All of a sudden, out of nowhere, she would burst into heinous laughter, a sickening, shrill cackle, as though something evil possessed her.

Papaw finally had mercy on me and stopped at a bus station somewhere midway. He bought me a ticket and called my parents to pick me up. I could tell by the helpless, pained look on his face as he put me on that bus, he had no idea what else to do!

That would be the last time I ever really spent any significant amount of time with my grandparents. Papaw had a couple of heart attacks before he died in 1978. Just like Mamaw, he was a heavy smoker. Although I would see her again on rare occasions over the rest of her life, for all intent and purposes, that trip was really when Mamaw died for me—in my heart.

A Search for Answers

My product training on neuroleptic drugs included education in the syndromes of psychosis and their treatments. This area greatly interested me because Mamaw had been diagnosed first with major depression, then with schizophrenia, then as bipolar, and, ultimately, with a schizoaffective disorder. She had been institutionalized, off and on, throughout her adult life. She responded poorly to treatment, and her condition deteriorated with time. This is known in psychiatry as the revolving door syndrome and is common in patients diagnosed with mental illness and treated with drugs.

Once, while institutionalized in a psychiatric ward, she obtained a knee injury from being wrestled to the floor by an attendant and then restrained. (She had gotten up in the middle of the night to get coffee.) The knee was operated on repeatedly and got infected. It never healed properly, and her leg eventually required amputation. She developed a severe case of buccalfacial tics and made gross lip-smacking and cud-chewing movements involuntarily with her mouth. I knew Mamaw had been on a variety of psychiatric drugs over the years, but I often wondered if this was the result of the Haldol she had taken.

Mamaw finally died of congestive heart failure at the age of seventy-nine. However, the grandmother I knew and loved was dead decades before they buried her body. I regret to say that I didn't even attend her funeral. I didn't know the woman being buried that day, and I had already mourned the loss of the one I had lost many years before that. Apparently, I wasn't the only one who felt that way. Mamaw's illness had taken its toll on the family overall. I was told a confrontation erupted when one of my mother's half-sisters emphatically remarked, "Let's plant her and get it over with!"

Her illness caused me such significant trauma as a child that I wanted desperately to understand her disease. In addition to that, there had been an ongoing dispute between family members for years about whether her medications and treatments were helping or hurting her. Opinions on this subject were passionately heated and divided. My mother was adamant the drugs seemed to make Mamaw worse:

> It was apparent by her speech alone that she had suffered brain damage. She sounded mentally retarded when she talked!

My aunts sided with the doctors. Mamaw would only get worse without her medication! Ultimately, I just wanted to know the truth. An underlying current of fear was growing in me that I carried some "defective gene" that would eventually make me "crazy" like Mamaw. Perhaps it was a premonition of things to come.

(It should be noted that schizoaffective disorder is characterized by chronic psychotic symptoms and recurrent manic or depressive episodes. It is considered more severe and complicated than schizophrenia or bipolar illness. Treatment generally involves a more complex regimen of medications. Antidepressants often worsen the psychotic symptoms) (Drummond 127).

The Seeds of Sorrow: Gertrude's Story

My great-grandmother, the family matriarch, raised several of her grandchildren. I adored my great-grandmother, who had an endearing Southern drawl and a funny phraseology when she talked. She was also a cat lover that took in every stray kitty around. At times, nearly forty to fifty cats were living in the barn and on the hillside behind her house. Only a special few were allowed inside her house. She would feed them by lining up pie tins on the sidewalk out back, filling them with dry food and calling "kitty, kitty, kitty" as a sea of felines emerged from under the porch, around the house, out of the barn, and seemingly everywhere! My most poignant memories today are of the smell of Ivory soap in her bathroom and the taste of her chocolate chip cookies with 7-Up. I can easily conjure a mental image of me as a child, swinging my legs under her kitchen table while gobbling down the cookies. The big, floor radiator groaning and spitting as it fired itself up to produce heat.

My mother had lived with my great-grandmother, Mamaw Wheeler, from the time she was three years old until she married my father at the age of sixteen. Mom's biological father, Wayne Cole, was an alcoholic who had impregnated two women at the same time and married the other woman. He was never a significant part of my mother's life, and she would not meet him until she was an adult.

Wayne Cole was an odd character. (He passed away some years ago.) The few times I saw him when I was young, he sort of frightened me. He had one arm that had been severed in an accident just below the elbow. He never wore a prosthesis that I knew of. On the other hand, his hairdo, slicked back with pomade, and a thick hillbilly dialect made him kind of funny. Still, I could sense a deep wounding suffered by my mother because of his abandonment. For that reason, I refused to like him.

My grandmother married my mother's stepfather, Junie, who had a quick temper when he was young. He was said to have been abusive to my mom. So, Mom was sent to live in Kentucky with Mamaw Wheeler, or as my mother called her, "Mom Wheeler". (She would always refer to her biological mother as *Mother*.)

Mamaw Wheeler married several times following the tragic death of my grandmother's father, who was accidentally shot by his own father when she was only five years old. Subsequently, a couple of the men Mamaw Wheeler married were explosive, mean alcoholics. One even tried to burn down their house when my mother was a small child. The only one of these men I would ever know, Cecil Wheeler, lived in the unfinished basement of the house and never came up to the living area. Apparently, he was banished to the basement to live several years before because of his drunken behavior. Even after he stopped drinking, he decided he would stay there. I never questioned the oddity of that arrangement until I was much older. There were so many unique aspects about my family and its history. That little tidbit seemed negligible.

Mamaw Wheeler had also raised my great-uncle's children, Nina, Sam, and Alvin. That was the first family funeral I ever attended. Their father, Jennings, ended his own life by eating a revolver. He was said to have suffered from PTSD, severely depressed following WWII, as did his younger brother, Glen, who eventually died of alcoholism. The children's mother, Thelma (no relation by blood) had a nervous breakdown following her husband's suicide. She was institutionalized. None of these second cousins would fare well as adults. All suffered from serious psychological problems and/or drug and alcohol addictions.

My great-grandmother's only offspring that appeared to be normal was my Great-Aunt Kathleen. However, I can't help but wonder if her youthful wild rebellion, promiscuity, and party-girl reputation didn't stem from alcohol and drug use, and if perhaps her recreational drug use wasn't an attempt to stabilize her moods. Kathleen was known by other family members to still use marijuana late in life. Witty, fun, and youthfully spirited to this day, she remains one of my favorite relatives.

8

The Genetic Theory of Mental Illness

"There probably exists in the mental life of the individual not only what he has experienced himself, but...an archaic heritage...The archaic heritage includes not only dispositions, but also ideational contents, memory traces of the experience of former generations."

—Sigmund Freud, *Moses and Monotheism*

In his book, *Blaming the Brain*, Dr. Elliot Valenstein says:

> Genes are responsible for establishing the scaffolding or fundamental organization of the brain, but a large amount of the neuronal growth that leads to the establishment of connections has been shown to be influenced (if not guided) by experience. There is no way that the one hundred thousand genes in the human genome could determine the precise configuration of the estimated 10 trillion synaptic connections in the human brain.

He further explains that biochemical and other biological changes in the brain may be the result of a patient's mental and behavioral state. Therefore, it cannot be assumed that any "biological marker" found in patients with a particular mental disorder is the cause of that disorder (Valenstein 144).

Genes do not necessarily determine our destiny. When it comes to behavior, it would be highly unlikely that any single gene could be responsible for mood instability. For example, if one parent is bipolar, there is still less than a twenty percent chance that the children will develop the disorder. Natural selection will generally weed out major genetic defects, and this does not prove to be the case in mental illness. Our attachment in infancy, the kind of nurturing we receive, the trauma we sustain, and how we are impacted by others in childhood remain an important part of how we adapt to our environment and stress our entire lives (Whybrow 258).

Richard Lewontin, an outspoken critic of the exaggerated claims made in genetic studies, is a renowned geneticist and Harvard professor who wrote *Biology as Ideology*. In it, he says:

> The fact is, not a single study of personality traits in human populations successfully disentangles similarity because of shared family experience and similarity because of genes...The argument confuses the observation [that a condition is running in families] with its explanation (Glenmullen 199).

Consider the evidence that schizophrenia and depression, especially manic depression, tends to run in families. (Mine is a prime example.) This alone is not proof of a genetic cause because poverty also runs in families. However, strong epidemiological evidence also supports the inheritance factor in mental disorders and is substantiated by studies comparing twins and data obtained from studies of adopted children (Valenstein 144–145).

Although no reports to date of the discovery of a gene responsible for manic-depressive disorders or schizophrenia have replicated, most knowledgeable people are convinced there is sufficient evidence to suggest genetic factors play some role in the etiology (origin) of mental disorders. Therefore, it is reasonable to assume people may inherit a predisposition to develop mental disorders. Valenstein uses the term *diathesis*, which originally comes from pathology. It means there is a constitutional predisposition or tendency toward developing a particular disease, but that predisposition is only realized under specific conditions (Valenstein 145).

In the case of my family, it appeared that stress, genetic predisposition, and learning and social networks had all played a part in determining our vulnerability to depression and bipolar disorder. But I certainly couldn't help but wonder if the final element that precipitated each illness had not been our exposure to potent, CNS-altering drugs. After all, it does not require a broken brain to respond negatively to drugs. Many psychoactive substances produce profound effects on the brains of people who have nothing wrong with them. Ask anyone who has smoked a joint, snorted a line of cocaine, taken a shot of tequila, or drank a cup of espresso. These drugs pretty much affect everyone—to varying degrees—in the same way (Breggin, *Talking Back to Prozac*, 37).

Linking Bipolar Illness to an Endocrine Disorder

My last full-time position (before becoming an independent contractor) was as a cardiovascular and diabetes specialist rep with Bristol-Myers Squibb. I was there for the beginning of the cholesterol wars selling Pravachol (pravastatin). I also helped educate America about the silent killer aspect of hypertension with the ace-inhibitors, Capoten (captopril) and Monopril (fosinopril). I witnessed the onslaught of the diabetes epidemic that has now swept the United States while selling Glucophage (metformin). I profited from the ill-fated diabetes drug, Rezulin, that was fast-tracked through the FDA in six months, only to be pulled off the market later because of several deaths that resulted from liver failure.

Interestingly enough, I had heard immediate concerns expressed by specialists in the field about this drug. They were all talking about an editorial that had appeared in the *New England Journal of Medicine* discussing liver failure. Regardless, Rezulin was a tremendous marketing success. In a bid for the lucrative pre-diabetic market, reps even told doctors it could *prevent* diabetes. Millions of patients were placed on Rezulin in a matter of months. Warner-Lambert reluctantly announced the removal of Rezulin from the American market in March 2000, almost thirty months after the first reports of liver failure had surfaced. Great Britain had withdrawn it from their market in December 1997. All in all, Rezulin would be suspected in 391 deaths and linked to 400 cases of liver failure. However, in spite of the rocky ride, Rezulin managed to generate $2.1 billion in annual sales before its demise (Strand 67-71).

In my training to sell and compete in these highly competitive markets, I learned a lot about blood sugar, blood pressure, the adrenals, and the role cortisol plays in hormonal regulation. I put this information to use in my own hypothesis about my family mental illness. As I tracked the history of bipolar illness specifically, several things became very clear. One was that there was definitely an endocrine component to this illness because it surfaced in times of peak pituitary activity in our lives, for example, in the teens, postpartum, and perimenopausal years. The cyclic nature of the female hormonal cycle itself mimics the fluctuations of the illness. Mood is closely linked to hormones.

Neurons are very sensitive to their hormonal environment. The hormones produced by stress, particularly cortisol and thyroxin, can be key influences in determining the limbic brain's (the part of the brain that experiences feeling and controls mood) homeostasis (balance). Any rapid changes in hormone levels require the brain to make immediate adjustments and can result in unstable mood changes while adaptation occurs (Whybrow 212). Chronic arousal of the limbic brain induced by stress can lead to a process called *kindling*. Stress kindles the activity of neurons, much in the way a fire is kindled. Kindling can be thought of as aberrant, learned activity by the brain and indicates a sensitization to stimulation. In experiments done on animals with cocaine, the kindling was capable of "initiating long-lasting, possibly permanent changes in neuronal excitement" (Whybrow 166). Prolonged or repeated stress through "this kindling mechanism may have the capacity to modify the long-term genetic expression of behavior" (Whybrow 188). Chronic stress can result in a hyperactive cortisol response and cause "anxiety, insomnia, exhaustion, and disruption of function until a vicious feedback cycle develop" (Whybrow 167).

Secondly, our brain's homoeostasis is further interrupted by the introduction of CNS-altering exogenous chemicals, for example, drugs and alcohol. It produces excess serotonin to compensate for the damaged neurotransmitters. The rise and fall of the chemical levels creates the classic mood swings experienced as manic-depressive episodes. This hypersensitivity to various drugs and substances was an obvious inherited factor that linked our mental illnesses to a possible biologic predisposition.

You cannot separate the effects of chemicals on the body from the brain. When the bloodstream is full of chemicals, they will interfere with brain functioning. Many of the depressive episodes I tracked were a direct result of anesthesia administered with childbirth or for other surgical procedures. (In fact, I recently had a hypomanic reaction when given Versed, a very short-acting benzodiazepine that was used in my anesthesia, and Restoril, another benzodiazepine I was prescribed as a sleep aid following minor cosmetic surgery.) Others' symptoms were directly related to the administration of antidepressants, stimulants, pain medication, or other mind-altering drugs that were prescribed following some stressful life event such as an accident, divorce, death, or postwar experience. Many of us had experienced repetitive adverse drug reactions throughout our lifetimes.

Nearly everyone who suffered from bipolar illness and/or depression in my family had glycemic (blood sugar) issues. Most were hypoglycemic initially. Some became diabetic with time because hypoglycemia is a predisposing factor to developing diabetes. I, myself, had gestational diabetes with my pregnancy, but I would battle with hypoglycemia thereafter. Even the alcoholism in my lineage could be linked to blood sugar issues.

The brain will create cravings for glucose (sugar) when it is in crisis. Blood glucose is the main fuel of the brain and is critical in regulating its activity. If the brain is low or runs out of fuel, brain cells begin to die. As a preservation technique, you can develop cravings for sugary food or alcohol, which is nearly one hundred percent sugar, as a sort of jump-start for the brain. We had all experienced cravings for sugar and/or alcohol.

The first endocrine organ to come into contact with ingested chemicals is the pancreas. The pancreas, under attack from the chemical toxicity, misinterprets the stimuli and produces insulin. The extra insulin in the blood then lowers the blood sugar level excessively, and the brain puts out distress signals to the adrenals to release adrenaline (and cortisol) in order to convert glycogen into glucose and increase blood sugar. We often consume substances like alcohol, caffeine, nicotine, or sugary snacks in order to achieve that equivalent of the adrenaline rush and spike the blood sugar. However, this behavior creates additional problems by dropping blood sugar levels even lower than before, thus perpetuating a vicious cycle. If the progress of disease is not halted by severe dietary and/or lifestyle changes, the pancreas eventually burns out and diabetes is the result.

The list of hypoglycemic symptoms is strikingly similar to bipolar symptoms as well as serotonin toxicity. *Taber's Medical Dictionary* lists hypoglycemic symptoms in their order of frequency:

> exhaustion, depression, insomnia, anxiety, irritability, headaches, vertigo, sweating, tremor (internal trembling), tachycardia (palpitation of heart), muscle pain and backache, anorexia, crying spells, phobias, difficulty in concentration, numbness, chronic indigestion, mental confusion, cold hands or feet, blurred vision, muscular twitching or abdominal spasms, fainting or blackouts, convulsions, and suicidal tendencies (Tracy 331).

Tempers flair easily in individuals with blood sugar imbalances, and the alcoholics in my family all have a tendency toward violence and explosive temperaments when intoxicated. This has landed many of them in trouble with the law. Most confessed to having blackouts or severe memory loss after drinking excessively. Several reported severe moodiness if they skip meals.

I became convinced this "mental illness" and "alcoholism" that runs in my family has a much larger physiological component than was given credit or consideration by our doctors. Granted, our family history is as stressful and dysfunctional as they come, which would substantiate an experiential or psychological component to our illnesses. But if there was a biochemical imbalance to be blamed for our collective issues of criminality, drug abuse, alcoholism, depression, and other behavioral abnormalities, it did not appear to be a brain defect to me. Instead, it appeared to be an endocrine defect that was passed from generation to generation. After evaluating all the predisposing factors, it was amazing to me that any of us had escaped the sanitarium considering the onslaught of chemicals we are exposed to in our environment and the poor nutrition plaguing our modern culture.

Orthomolecular Psychiatry: Feeding the Brain

It was validating to discover that several researchers had indeed postulated there was a correlation between mental disorders and endocrine deficiencies or blood sugar imbalances. There is substantial documentation that delinquent probationers who are placed on restricted diets to control the intake of processed foods, sugar, caffeine, and other additives and who increase the consumption of fresh fruits and vegetables have remarkable improvements in behavior and attitude.

Similar results have been obtained with schizophrenic and bipolar patients who were previously unresponsive to medication. Food that feeds the brain and allows the rich neuronal environment needed for proper brain transmission and communication has an ameliorating effect on attitude and behavior. If the diet contains the substances needed for proper brain function, it works normally. Behavior is then both rational and constructive. A healthy body means a healthy mind. However, if the brain does not receive the proper nutrients and in addition is struggling to overcome drug toxicity, it will malfunction. Anything from irritability to psychosis can result. This is the foundation of orthomolecular psychiatry, the restoration of the proper molecular balance of the brain. This dietary approach is generally accompanied by vitamin and mineral supplementation and/ or other therapies such as counseling (Reed Stitt 75, 137).

Orthomolecular psychiatry has gotten very little attention in the field. No wonder, it is relatively uncomplicated theoretically. It doesn't cost a lot of money and require a tremendous amount of technology or specialized staff. It is not profitable at all to industry. Therefore, it has remained a back alley approach basically ignored by the scientific community. The most wonderful thing about the orthomolecular approach is that it is completely safe compared to drug therapy. No one has died or had permanent brain damage from eating healthfully. In addition, many young people whose lives were destined to be wasted away in the correctional system have since become productive, contributing members of society (Reed Stitt 135).

Additionally, in 1999, a study was published in the *American Journal of Psychiatry* clearly substantiating previous theories about the "disturbance in glucose homeostasis in psychiatric populations." The study states there was an, "elevated frequency of diabetes mellitus in hospitalized manic-depressive patients" (Cassidy et al).

What Causes Manic Psychosis?

It has been scientifically proven that experience can modify brain anatomy, causing structural and functional changes in the brain. Numerous experiments have shown exposure to stressful situations, for example, can produce long-lasting brain changes. Animals that are stressed continually have a hypersensitive response to amphetamines, even when the drugs are administered months later. Stress can produce changes in the same class of dopamine neurons on which the neuroleptic drugs act. Even when the dopamine neurons that have been removed from the brains of stressed animals are challenged with amphetamines in a petri dish, excessive amounts of dopamine are released. These results indicate that stress can produce prolonged physical changes in dopamine neurons that make them hypersensitive not only to drugs, but also to subsequent stress (Valenstein 127).

It is important to be aware that a number of drugs, both legal and illegal, can induce psychotic symptoms. Among these are steroids, stimulants (for example, ephedra, diet pills, and antidepressants), amphetamines, cocaine, hallucinogens (such as ecstasy, mescaline, peyote, mushrooms, and LSD), hypnotic painkillers and sleep aids (like Halcion, Vicodin, and Oxycontin), marijuana, and PCP. Psychosis has also been reported in rare instances with the antibiotic class known as quinolones. Stephen Fried, an investigative journalist and husband of a "Floxie" (Floxin victim) details his own wife's life-altering adverse drug reaction to Floxin (ofloxacin) in his sobering book *Bitter Pills*. Fried's wife, who took only one dose of this powerful antibiotic for a minor urinary tract infection, now permanently suffers from a drug-induced manic-depressive illness and was told she must take mood stabilizers and antipsychotic drugs for the rest of her life.

Drugs can become neurotoxic when they reach high enough concentrations to penetrate the blood-brain barrier. Drug-induced manic psychosis is a severe psychotic disorder whose symptoms include insomnia, extreme overactivity, racing thoughts, grandiosity, paranoia, exhausting outbursts of energy and suicide (Breggin and Cohen 62). Psychosis can also occur in bipolar disorder, depression, dementia, and post-traumatic stress disorder. This makes the appropriate diagnosis of psychotic symptoms and identification of adverse drug reactions extremely critical to the patient's treatment and recovery. And, because there is no objective measure to prove or disprove a patient has any psychiatric disorder, this can be a difficult assessment, even for the well-trained psychiatrist (Drummond 35).

Acute psychosis is generally a response to stressful situations or, as I said, can sometimes follow the use of stimulants, psychoactive drugs, or prolonged use of marijuana. It is imperative to immediately discontinue the use of any drug that causes psychotic symptoms. This type of psychosis is known as brief reactive psychosis and generally abates within the time necessary to detoxify the body from the offending chemicals. People normally return to their usual ability to function once their symptoms subside, although permanent brain damage can occur (Drummond 124).

Neuroleptics: A Combination Chemical Straight Jacket and Lobotomy

One medication class used to treat psychosis and schizophrenia is known as neuroleptics or antipsychotics. The term neuroleptic essentially describes what these drugs do, that is, they "clamp down, in the manner of a chemical restraint, on the central nervous system" (Whitaker 208). They can dramatically curb the neurotransmitter activity that underlies motor movement. Neuroleptics alter behavior and thinking by partially shutting down dopamine receptor pathways, in essence, having the effect of a chemical lobotomy. These drugs cause a variety of unpleasant side effects, including weight gain, emotional blunting, fatigue, visual disturbances, constipation, urinary retention, sexual dysfunction, and dry mouth. However, the most alarming side effects associated with these drugs are the muscular side effects such as rigidity, decreased muscle movement, tremor, muscle spasms, and restlessness.

Moreover, neuroleptics can cause permanent neurological damage known as tardive dyskinesia. This is a devastating disorder involving abnormal, involuntary, constant, rhythmical muscle movements, commonly referred to as tics. These movements generally affect the mouth, tongue, hands, fingers, trunk of the body, and toes. Mouth movements can mimic the action of chewing gum, or the tongue may involuntarily dart out of the mouth, also known as fly tongue. Trunk movements may appear as constant rocking back and forth. In severe cases, body parts may lock in bizarre positions.

Women, the elderly, and people with brain injury are more likely to develop tardive dyskinesia. There is no cure for it, but there is a ten to thirty percent chance of developing it if you take an antipsychotic drug for more than one year (Drummond 122).

For political and financial reasons, most of the research in psychiatry has been done on white males. In 1977, the FDA issued guidelines that practically banned "women of child-bearing potential" from early clinical trials (Phase I and Phase II). These trials generally determine a drug's standard dosage. They also determine the baseline of a drug's toxicity. So, by law, these studies have only been populated by men (Fried 265). The absence of research in other populations has led the medical and psychiatric professions to make treatment recommendations by extrapolating findings made from these adult white male studies. Consequently, the unique biological makeup of women and other groups is not taken into account, and psychiatric medications (among others) can pose additional risk to these patients (Drummond 34). It is also important to remember that clinical trials done during the approval process for drugs involve healthy subjects or patients that only have the disease being studied. The participants are rarely allowed to be on concomitant drug therapies. This is not the case in the general population and the real world (Strand 109).

It is a travesty that neuroleptics are some of the most frequently prescribed drugs in mental hospitals and are widely used in board and care homes, nursing homes, institutions for people with mental retardation, children's facilities, and prisons. These drugs are also given to millions of patients in public clinics and dispensed to hundreds of thousands of people in private psychiatric practices. Some of the symptoms for which they are prescribed are off-label indications such as anxiety and sleep disturbance. All too often, they are administered to children with emotional and behavioral problems, even children living at home and going to school (Breggin, *Toxic Psychiatry*, 51).

You may recall the outrage among Americans in the 1970s when Soviet dissidents revealed they had been tortured by the KGB with mind control drugs that completely destroyed their will to live and left them brain-damaged, psychotic, or delusional. At a 1971 disarmament conference in East Berlin, the consensus was that "psychotoxins were weapons directed against the further existence of an independently thinking and acting society." The World Psychiatric Association further condemned the Soviet Union for the use of neuroleptics in Soviet dissidents in 1977, saying the practice amounted to nothing less than a combination of lobotomies and torture ("Forced Drugging"). The drug that was frequently used in that torture was the neuroleptic I sold, Haldol.

The neuroleptics are the main constituents contained in tranquilizer darts and the injections used by veterinarians in subduing vicious animals. By impairing the limbic system, the arousal response is blunted, thereby tranquilizing the animal. Veterinary literature and practice has established these drugs must be limited to short-term use only. They are considered to be very dangerous to animals, even though it is often more difficult to produce the permanent drug-induced neurological disorders in animals than it is in humans. Why then would American psychiatrists presume them to be any safer in people?

The bottom line is that important aspects of the psychiatric treatment of women, children, elderly, and other ethnic groups have yet to be adequately studied. So, the side effects of these drugs that are specific to them are generally unknown.

Dr. Peter Breggin sums up his position on the use of neuroleptic drugs quite profoundly in his book entitled *Toxic Psychiatry*:

> Despite the best efforts, we can never fully anticipate all of the damaging effects inflicted on the individual by the neuroleptics and other toxic drugs. We must assume that numerous harmful effects go unnoticed. There is an analogy here to environmental pollution, where likewise we can notice, measure, and anticipate only the most obviously damaging effects. By the time we do become aware of new dangers, we've already done an unconscionable amount of harm and for the health of many people, it's too late (91).

Atypical Antipsychotics: One Man's Trash Is Another Man's Treasure

If there is anywhere that the scientific background of psychiatric drugs is questionable, it is with the atypical antipsychotics. Once again, the industry created a new name for the newer drugs to divert the negative publicity now associated with neuroleptic-induced tardive dyskinesia. Unfortunately, the atypical antipsychotics have also been found to cause many of the same side effects as the older neuroleptic drugs, including tardive dyskinesia.

At least the neuroleptics are pretty much seen for what they are, chemical restraints for combative, psychotic patients. However, the atypical antipsychotics are touted as breakthrough drugs and as a more advanced treatment option. They are also promoted as having fewer side effects and better outcomes that help schizophrenics lead more functional lives. I have talked to patients who say they are doing well on them, but a review of the scientific facts brings to light serious concerns.

One of the saddest elements of this story I uncovered was how the patients in these atypical drugs' clinical trials were selected and treated. Robert Whitaker reveals the shocking history and continuing mistreatment of our mentally ill in his book, *Mad in America*. Among the many injustices committed against these poor souls were the clinical protocols that required patients to be abruptly withdrawn from their existing medications. The abrupt withdrawal was expected to exacerbate psychotic hallucinations and delusions. However, as Whitaker notes:

> Abrupt withdrawal (as opposed to gradual withdrawal as we've already learned) is also known to put patients at risk of severe clinical deterioration.

It is contrary to good clinical practice, and it increases the risk of suicide, which is precisely how many people died in the trials (270).

All told, seven people killed themselves in the Serlect (sertindole) clinical trials, another atypical that was launched in Europe in 1996 but later withdrawn because of cardiac side effects in 1997. Serlect was never approved in the United States. At least ten patients committed suicide in the Risperdal trials, fifteen in the Zyprexa studies, and four in the Seroquel (quetiapine) experiments. Even more appalling is the fact that when the trial results for these drugs were reported in the scientific journals, they completely excluded the loss of life that had occurred (Whitaker 272). Most of these patients had gone seeking help from their doctors and, instead, had been put at grave risk, treated like ordinary guinea pigs or lab rats for pharmaceutical research purposes!

FDA reviewers reportedly scoffed at the data submitted by Janssen and Eli Lilly during their face-off wars between Risperdal (risperidone) and Zyprexa (olanzapine) and pointed out how the manufacturers had biased the trial designs in order to produce superior results over the older neuroleptics. In fact, following the review of the first three atypicals, the FDA did not find any convincing evidence the atypicals were any more effective than the existing treatments. However, it is not necessary to prove superiority over existing therapies to win FDA approval for a drug. It is only necessary to show superiority over placebo. The manufacturers' attempts to show superiority over older, less expensive neuroleptics was a marketing ploy to gain market share for the newer drugs which sold for ten to thirty times the price of the older ones (Whitaker 282).

Use of the newer atypical antipsychotics has been linked to dramatic increases in triglycerides and the development of diabetes. This prompted a joint warning about these drugs to be issued by the American Diabetes Association, American Psychiatric Association, North American Association for the Study of Obesity, and American Association of Clinical Endocrinologists ("Risks of Anti-Psychotic Drugs Eyed").

Additionally, on April 11, 2005, the FDA issued a public health advisory alerting health care providers, patients, and caregivers to safety concerns regarding the off-label uses of atypical antipsychotics. The FDA's statement said the treatment of behavioral issues in elderly patients with atypical antipsychotics had been associated with increased mortality in this population, and that clinical studies had substantiated a higher death rate associated with their use in geriatrics (U.S. Food 2005d).

So, even if some patients do receive a perceived benefit from the newer atypicals, there is the added risk that overall health may be negatively impacted, leading to additional medical complications or early death for many. All of these things must be factored into the risk-to-benefit ratio when assessing the true value of the atypical antipsychotics.

Antipsychotic drugs do not knowingly fix any brain abnormalities or balance any brain chemicals. What they do is suppress brain function in a manner that restrains physical mobility and diminishes certain psychotic symptoms. Like neuroleptics, these drugs grossly affect dopamine levels in the brain, a situation which is known to increase some people's vulnerability to psychosis. Long-term outcomes with the use of any of the antipsychotics are dismal at best. The World Health Organization has reported the outcomes for psychiatric diagnoses to be much better in countries where these medications are not used or are used less frequently.

Regardless, total sales of antipsychotic drugs in 2004 grew in excess of ten percent year over year (IMS Health 2005a). Currently, sales of Zyprexa, Eli Lilly's atypical antipsychotic and newest and sweetest cash cow, have now surpassed sales of Prozac. (Although it went off patent in 2001, Prozac still brought in $559 million to the company coffers last year) (Swiatek). Despite stiff competition and the negative publicity from reports linking it to weight gain and diabetes, in 2004, Zyprexa sales ranked fifth in the top ten pharmaceutical products sold globally racking up a cool $4.8 billion in sales (IMS Health 2005b).

9

Crazy Just Like Your Mother: Dolores' Story

"Nothing has a stronger influence psychologically on their children than the unlived life of the parent."

—Carl G. Jung

"Mommy has a mental illness, just like Mamaw. It never goes away, and they don't know how to fix it." That's how my father explained it to me as a little girl as we sat talking for hours about our family trials and tribulations. However, in my mind, that translated to "Mommy is *crazy* just like Mamaw." This was in no small part due to the fact that when they were fighting, my father repeatedly told my mother, "You *crazy* bitch!" He would snarl between clenched teeth, either unaware or unconcerned I was listening, "You're *crazy,* just like your mother!"

That particular explanation did nothing to quell my fears or make it any easier for me to cope with the tremendous mood swings my mother would have and the resulting chaos that would consume our household.

We were like a family of trapeze artists, never knowing which wrong step might send us plummeting to the ground below. In fact, I think the circus analogy is very appropriate for my family dynamics. Our lives were filled with adrenaline rushes and high drama. We were an organization of misfits, so to speak, that performed in front of audiences with polish and pizzazz. Just like in a circus, behind the scenes and after the show, abuses were taking place that were unknown to the outside world, suffered in silence by innocent captives.

The fights that would define my childhood sent me and my younger sister scampering to hide in closets. If my father had been drinking, the fighting was physical and violent, so we learned to take cover when things escalated. The chaotic noise coming from the hallway and bedrooms could be terrifying to the untrained ear. Furniture was overturned. Doors were slammed, and dishes crashed. We waited with bated breath until the crying, wailing, screaming, and cursing had stopped.

Sometimes, Mother would plead for help and beg us to call the police. On more than one occasion, I remember trying to live down the embarrassment at school of the police coming to our house. Everyone would know and be whispering about it the next day.

Following many of their fights, Dad would gather his things and head for a hotel for the night. Mom would eventually run out of steam and collapse, sobbing and exhausted on her bed. Only then would my sister and I venture out. We were like soldiers returning to the battlefield, surveying the damage and assisting the wounded. We were our mother's caretakers. We were always there to pick up the pieces of her shattered life.

I don't know when my parents' marriage went south, but they had traumatic fights from my earliest memories on. My mother was never officially diagnosed with any mental illness, although she was treated for her nerves more than once. It is impossible to know now which drugs she was given, but I would be shocked if she hadn't been given tricyclic antidepressants somewhere along the line. I do know she was given Valium.

Whatever it was she was given for her nerves initially made her sleep a lot. Eventually, it precipitated a cleaning frenzy that would last for days. There was a wild look in her eyes that I would later identify as mania, but, back then, I only knew that look meant trouble for me. Mother was on the warpath! Fortunately for her (and us), the SSRIs had not yet been discovered.

I recall a particularly difficult time in 1969. I was ten, and my mother was twenty-nine. My Uncle Sonny had been killed in Vietnam. The funeral was a heart-wrenching display of raw emotion and grief. I had been asked to sing and was directed to stand behind the coffin. A curtain separated me from the congregation. I had a side view of the casket, but I could not see the audience. My knees trembled as the music began, and I felt faint from the heat. It was almost impossible to sing as my emotions swelled and caught in my throat. My grandmother snapped during the service, got out of her seat, and approached the coffin. She started dumping the contents of her purse onto the glass that allowed us to view, but not touch, Sonny's body. (He had stepped on a mine and was missing body parts. Therefore, the casket was only halfway open and covered by glass.) She was searching for smelling salts she had been given while watching a neighbor's ailing dog.

In the days following her brother's burial, my mother's moods were erratic and volatile. She would lock herself in her bedroom for days crying. She would refuse to bathe, eat, or interact with anyone else. Sometimes, I would sit outside her door on the floor reading, just waiting to hear her stir or get up to use the bathroom. Other times, I would sit, gently consoling her through the door as she sobbed uncontrollably from the other side. I attempted to coax her out of the room or to let me come in. When she finally did open the door, the room was dark and dreary with all the drapes drawn and windows closed and stunk of body odor. Piles of books, magazines, and photos lay strewn about the bed amidst discarded snot-laden Kleenex. Mom lay curled up in a fetal position wearing her housecoat and pajamas, appearing almost comatose on the bed.

As the school bus approached the farm road to my house, I would begin feeling anxious in anticipation of what I might find. Leaving Mom in one frame of mind that morning did not ensure you would encounter her in the same demeanor that afternoon. It was a crapshoot at any given time, but it was especially brutal that particular year.

This scene would repeat itself over and over again as I grew up. The family would literally walk on eggshells during these episodes, fearing anything one said or did could set Mom off! Eventually, I started losing compassion for my mother and closed my heart to the abuse perpetrated against her by my father. Part of me felt like she deserved it. She often started the fights! Part of me even cheered in retaliation when he blackened her eye or hurt her in some other way. However, I later realized that was my own coping mechanism to survive the psychological pain she had inflicted on me. Sometimes, it is easier to hate your abusers than it is to justify loving them.

Growing up with Dr. Jekyll and Mr. Hyde

Probably the most difficult part of bipolar disorder for a child to accept and assimilate is living with the two faces of Dr. Jekyll and Mr. Hyde. A child with a bipolar parent experiences life much like a roller coaster ride. There are alternating highs and lows that either thrill and elate you or scare you half to death! When my mother was hypomanic or in the initial stages of mania, her moods were childlike and free-spirited. She was so young to begin with, but, even so, she still appeared exceptionally youthful. An unlived childhood beckoned her to romp and play carefree as an adult. We would ride in her VW bug with the top down and the wind in our hair as the radio blared loudly.

I distinctly remember the immense sense of pride I felt about my beautiful mother when I was younger. She had long, thick, auburn hair and lovely blue-gray eyes. She also had a great sense of style and was always sporting the latest haircut and clothing design. Her gregarious, outgoing personality, coupled with an infectiously loud laugh, made her great fun during those times. Mom was intelligent, witty, and charming. She was a good cook and a phenomenal hostess.

Because of these qualities, she collected a cadre of friends over the years. I loved to daydream with Mom because she lived large in her dreams. She had an inquisitive, naïvety for her years and a spunky, determined outlook on life when she was consumed by grandiose ideas, usually her latest business venture that would be started in a flurry of hypomanic energy and then abandoned midstream when the dark clouds rolled back in.

These were the times I loved most, when we talked and laughed for hours on end and shopped until we dropped. Mom felt more like my friend than a parent, more like she does today. When Mom isn't depressed or agitated, I would still rather exchange ideas and talk with her more than anyone else I know. For example, while I was writing this book, she was a constant source of information and discourse on the subject matter, although much of what was written was an unflattering reminder of her former self and quite painful for her to read and relive.

This same lost childhood made Mom determined to give me all the experiences and opportunities that she had not had. To that end, I took tap dance, ballet, and piano lessons. I played French horn in the band and was a member of the "Sparkettes," my high school drill team. I also performed before local civic groups singing and reciting poetry. I was in choir and Job's Daughters. I participated in theatre and drama projects at school, and I won several local beauty pageants. Mom would also encourage me to be a foreign exchange student my junior year in high school. All of these things were things my mother would have loved to do.

Needless to say, not being mature enough to understand her motivations at the time, I started to resent Mom for what I saw as her attempts to live through me. As an adolescent, I pushed for greater autonomy and independence, and she felt threatened and abandoned. Of course, that only escalated the tension between us. When the histrionics would start consuming my life again, I could barely muster the tender feelings of love and pride I had felt so intensely for her before. She would nearly always beg for forgiveness following our fallouts, dissolving into emotional tears that would often melt my angry heart. By the time I left home, I had little compassion remaining. I simply could not integrate the dualism. Of course, my father's cruel response to Mom's agitation and depression only added fuel to the fire of her despair. I couldn't stand it any longer!

Ironically, as I was learning to speak Spanish, I discovered my mother's name in its exact spelling…D-O-L-O-R-E-S…translates to pain, sorrow and grief. It was almost as if her given name had eerily foretold her future.

Please, Don't Tell Anyone: Living with Shameful Family Secrets

My mother was an avid member of the local Women's Democrats. We had just come from a meeting. It was late when we dropped off my Aunt Phyllis, my dad's younger sister, at her house in Marion and headed back to Greentown. The house was unusually dark when we arrived home. I had to squint, straining my eyes to focus in the pitch-black darkness as Mom and I entered the family room from the garage. After my vision had adjusted, I could see my dad sitting at the kitchen table in his white boxer shorts and T-shirt. Illuminated by the moonlight streaming through the window, he was almost glowing in contrast. A half-empty, uncapped bottle of vodka sat on the table in front of him. My body stiffened in anticipation as I realized he had been drinking. It was one thing if Dad had a beer or two, but hard liquor always meant trouble!

"Where the hell have you been?" he demanded, slurring his speech.

"You're drunk, Arthur J," Mom retorted in disgust as she stubbornly and defiantly brushed past him and headed toward the hallway.

That's when I saw a faint gleam of light flash off the blade of the butcher knife Dad held in his hand. As he rose from behind the table to follow her, I completely froze up. Without warning, he lunged, grabbing her from behind. He was holding her in a choke hold in the crook of his left elbow with the blade of the knife pressed up against her throat as Mom begged and pleaded for him to let her go.

"Don't hurt me, Art…please, don't hurt me…you're drunk," she whimpered as she gasped for air and attempted to pry his arm lose.

"Oh, ain't you perty with your hair all done up and your war paint on?" he cajoled in a mocking tone.

"But you ain't nothin' but a slut, are you, Dee? Speak up…who you been out whorin' with?" he demanded between gritted teeth.

Then I remember hearing an unidentifiable sort of ripping sound. Once again, I saw a flash of light reflect from the knife as Dad abruptly jerked his right arm in an upward, sweeping motion. Not knowing what had just happened, I stood paralyzed, helplessly watching and half-expecting to see blood gush forth from my mother's severed throat! Instead, I watched as the silk scarf she had worn tied around her neck, which was fashionable in the 1960s, fell silently to the carpet below. Mom collapsed in a sobbing heap as Dad shoved her violently to the floor and then walked away. He had not even spoken to me or acknowledged my presence.

Suddenly, I remembered Michelle, who was a toddler at the time and had stayed home with my dad. My heart raced as I sprinted down the hallway to her bedroom. I threw open the door in anticipation. Thank God, there she lay, peacefully asleep and oblivious to the ordeal I had just witnessed. And thank God I did…for Dad not having hurt my mother this time, at least physically. I gently closed the door to Michelle's room with a sigh of relief as I heard the car spitting up gravel as Dad angrily backed down the driveway to leave. Then I headed back to the family room to comfort my mother.

Post-Traumatic Stress Disorder (PTSD)

Any witness to violence is a victim of violence. In June 1990, the *New York Times* reported on a study that found one traumatic experience that makes a person feel totally powerless can be enough to permanently alter their brain chemistry. The result is called post-traumatic stress disorder (PTSD). Children are especially vulnerable to PTSD because of their limited coping skills and inability to integrate the horror of trauma.

During such experiences, there is a tremendous surge of adrenaline, what is commonly referred to as the fight-or-flight syndrome. This is our body's natural alarm system that alerts us when it is necessary to flee or fight for our survival. It is controlled by the limbic system of the brain. Additionally, endorphins (hormones) are released to ease pain and assist in memory formation. A cellular imprint is then made upon the brain in order for it to remember the life-threatening circumstance. This keeps the brain from being caught off guard again in the future and can precipitate a continual state of hypervigilance or constant anxiety (Bradshaw 157). I often jokingly refer to this feeling as having my accelerator stuck. Believe me though, when it's happening, it is no laughing matter!

The most common symptom of PTSD is kindling. You will recall that kindling is the phenomenon that occurs when minor stressors, either negative or positive, cause an unpleasant arousal and increase in the release of norepinephrine and cortisol. This may further trigger panic attacks, mood irritability, fright, and insomnia. If the arousal is chronic, it can create symptoms of avoidance, social withdrawal, isolation, and depression. Each time a crisis situation has passed, the individual will have a hormonal withdrawal. This leads to additional symptoms such as restlessness, agitation, trembling, and other flu-like symptoms. Hence, the victim often becomes frightened again, which results in another hormonal surge. The kindling reoccurs, becoming a vicious cycle. People often try to self-medicate these unpleasant withdrawal symptoms with some form of addictive behavior or substance (Bradshaw 158).

10

The Era of Sex, Drugs, and Rock-and-Roll!

"Manic depression is touching my soul
I know what I want but I just don't know
How to go about getting' it
Feeling, sweet feeling
Drops from fingers, fingers
Manic depression is catchin' my soul…"

—Jimi Hendrix

My parents were really young compared to most of my classmates' parents, having married in their teens. Neither had a formal education past high school, and my dad spoke with a distinct, Appalachian drawl. Dad was a humorous, gentle-natured man who loved hunting and fishing. He didn't like crowds. In contrast to my mother, he wasn't much of a social butterfly. Unfortunately, like a lot of good 'ol boys, he had a mean streak when he drank. Both his father and younger brother were alcoholics. Dad had joined the United States Army when he turned eighteen. He was stationed in Germany when he came home on leave and met my mother at a roller skating rink in Ashland, Kentucky. They were both self-proclaimed graduates of the School of Hard Knocks, and they had left their clannish roots down south in search of employment and a brighter future together in the Midwest.

Born in 1959, I was at the tail end of the Baby Boomers. Growing up in the post-Vietnam war era, I had missed the heyday of the flower child and the call to unity, love, and peace that so deeply resonated to my soul. I loved Sonny and Cher, and I knew the words to every Beatles song. I wanted so badly to be a hippie, but I was too young!

No, mine would be the era of sex, drugs and rock-and-roll, a generation of apathetic souls caught up in the drama of their own little worlds who would choose to rebel, get stoned, and ignore society's problems rather than mobilize and do something about them. As a result, I would spend the majority of my adult life psychologically and/or physically dependent on drugs to escape my anger, pain, and symptoms of anxiety and depression.

That '70s Show, which is my favorite TV sitcom, so accurately depicts life as it was back then in the Midwest, including the cliquish group wars, the senseless pranks, and the youthful experimentation. In fact, I spent many hours in my own friends' basements passing doobies around as we discussed the latest piece of small-town gossip. Few of us knew or cared anything about world politics. Most of us had no aspirations to go to college or any career goals. The majority would either end up raising families and working in one of the local auto plants, Delco and Chrysler. Some would inherit responsibilities—and/or acreage—on their family farms. Our world pretty much ended at Indianapolis and Chicago, which was the furthest distance most of us had ever been away from home.

At school, I attempted to achieve my way out of my reality at home. I was constantly seeking the approval of my educators and adult mentors. I was an insatiable reader with a sharp mind and quick wit, a straight-A student, and a local beauty queen. My teachers liked me, but that didn't make me any more popular with my peers. They openly taunted my need for validation by the adult world.

When I won a scholarship to Brazil in 1976 as a foreign exchange student my junior year of high school, it was the opening of a whole new world to me. Brazilians were warm, hospitable people who had large, extended families and a true sense of community. I lived with a family of five in an apartment building in Sao Paulo. There were three teenage girls ages seventeen, sixteen, and thirteen—Maria Virginia, Maria Fernanda, and Maria Claudia. The oldest girl, Virginia, had been an exchange student herself and had just returned from Ohio. As is the custom, her family was reciprocating and housing a student from the United States. She spoke English fluently and quickly set about teaching me the Portuguese language.

I love to talk. I'm a Gemini. It's in my nature. So, in three month's time, I became fluent in Portuguese. I loved the Brazilian people and the beautiful country itself. I spent time on the beaches of Santos and in Rio de Janeiro. I saw the statue of Christ at Sugar Loaf Mountain, visited the northern state of Mato Grosso, and learned to traverse a foreign city of millions of people free from fear. Most importantly, I was received into the family unit and home of these wonderful people, as though I was one of their own. My Brazilian parents called me Maria Gwendolyn. For nine months, life was like a young girl's fantasy. Nobody knew about my past. They treated me like a princess, and I blossomed.

I attended a private, Catholic girl's school and hung out in exclusive country clubs and nightclubs with my sisters and their friends. Sometimes, Virginia would take me to campus with her. She had graduated high school and was studying elementary education at Mackenzie University in Sao Paulo. I loved the bohemian feel of the student body, the free and open forum of the classes, and the electric exchange of information and ideas between the teachers and the students. I knew then that I wanted to go to college.

When I returned to the United States during the second semester of my senior year, I was even more estranged from my peer group. A Brazilian student had come home with me to stay with us for six months, again the reciprocity rule of student exchange. She had been a friend of mine in Brazil, so we got along really well with one another. We would talk up a storm, of course, in Portuguese. Bell (short for Maria Isabel) didn't speak English very well, so I accommodated her in her own language. That didn't help me fit in any better with my classmates. Foreigners were looked down the nose at, just like they do Fes in *That '70s Show*. The fact we spoke a language nobody understood irked everybody else. I admit that it was rude, but we didn't mean to be rude. I found myself frequently defending my Brazilian student, and it placed an even wider rift between the locals and me.

All of my differences contributed to a torturous experience in school, where I was teased, ostracized, and gossiped about endlessly. It took me fifteen years before I would finally return to the scene of the crime for a class reunion. It took an additional ten before I would return once more and experience some closure and healing around that particular trauma in my life. Meg was the one who had encouraged me to attend my twenty-fifth class reunion. That road trip back to Greentown was one of the last carefree, fun times we would share together.

The need to succeed I had developed as a form of self-validation when I was a child would become an addiction later in life. Under the guise of accomplishment, a workaholic emerged. I used to think, because I was always busy, I was an accomplished, productive member of society. What I didn't realize was that I was running from my emotions, fears, and memories from childhood while using busy-ness (business) as my excuse to do so. I was afraid to stay idle for too long for fear my past would catch up with me. With little time left over for family and friendships, my life became all about my work. I would enjoy ten years of fast-track career success in industry before life came to a screeching halt and I collapsed, physically exhausted, depressed, and alone.

My point is, even given the best circumstances later in life (a good marriage, a lucrative career, a nice home, and so forth), one cannot run from the psychological repercussions of a traumatic childhood. The repressed pain haunts the psyche and manifests itself in the form of nightmares, depression, and obsessive-compulsive behavior at best. At worst, it develops into fits of anger and rage or other self-destructive behavior such as promiscuity and substance abuse.

A House Divided Cannot Stand

It really is not surprising that my sister, Michelle, and I have never been close. Besides the fact we were six years apart in age, Michelle's temperament is completely different from mine. She exhibited a quick, volatile temper very early in life. I, on the other hand, have always been a people pleaser. Fearing that expression of my anger would isolate me from others, I stuffed it down inside. Because of this, my father identified more closely with me than with my sister. When our parents fought, Dad would often take me and leave, separating the fight into two camps: theirs and ours.

I enjoyed these times alone with Dad. We would stop by the local grocery store and buy beanie-weenies, cheese and crackers, and a bottle of pop (as I called it back then). Then we would go sit by the reservoir and skip rocks while we ate and talked about God and Dad's philosophy on life.

Picture Andy Taylor (Griffith) as he would often instruct little Opie on life's deeper lessons. That TV character so closely resembled my father in his youth. Why, shucks, they even talked alike! Unfortunately, sometimes Dad's instructions to me were less than well-balanced.

"The man is the leader of his house. It says so in the Bible," he would say. "You should never challenge the authority of your husband! Even if you don't agree with him, he is the decision maker, and you should support him one hundred percent."

(What excellent advice that would turn out to be when both he and my mother later chastised me as an adult, for what they perceived as allowing my husband to manipulate and control me.) His talks would always end with the admonishment, "Don't ever be like your mother!"

Finally, after twenty-three years of fighting and dysfunction, my parents divorced. I was twenty at the time and a junior at Indiana University in Bloomington. Michelle was fourteen years old and a freshman in high school still living at home. This time, she would be the only one there to bear the brunt of my mother's emotional storm. I can only imagine what she went through!

Surprisingly, I was devastated by my parents' divorce. Even though our household had been so turbulent, it was all that I knew. I felt like the foundation of my very life had been swept away, and I was supposedly a full-grown adult at the time! For the first time, it hit me that I no longer had a home to go home to. I was on my own. This feeling would later help me as a child advocate to identify with children removed from their homes for neglect and abuse that, even though their lives were painfully dysfunctional at home, would cling to their parents and abusers out of fear of the unknown. It never occurred to them that there was something better than what they were living.

I think my mother resented my admiration for my father because our relationship was so crippled emotionally. She saw him for who he was in totality. I, on the other hand, idealized my dad. To me, he was a wise, compassionate, funny, brave, noble man who loved and feared God. I still saw him through the eyes of a child back then. He was my hero, my protectorate, my stability, and my security!

During their divorce, my mother would abruptly remove the veil of that illusion when she and a friend followed my father and his mistress to a local motel. Mom listened as my dad and his girlfriend had their interlude in an adjacent room. Thank God, I don't remember all the details because I was so freaked out by the story as she recounted it that I nearly lost consciousness. I remember the room spinning amidst the sound of her mockery, moaning, and laughing. I wanted to run. I wanted to burst out the door and never look back! I was sick, angry, and disgusted! I was angry at my father for his deception and lies, for pretending to be something he was not. I was angry at my mother for exposing me to this mental and emotional anguish. I was disgusted with them both.

I ended up taking Mom to the emergency room that night because she thought she was having a heart attack. Fortunately, it was only a panic attack, but the episode scared me enough and angered me to the extent that it was a defining moment in my growth process. Not only had my family structure disintegrated, but I had been completely debased spiritually as well. Everything Dad had taught me about God—everything about morality and what was right and what was wrong—now all came into question. Life seemed like a sick joke, and I felt betrayed, alone, and adrift in the world. So much for my happy ending!

Cross-Generational Bonding

When parents cross generation lines by sharing secrets or dividing the loyalty of children against other members of the family, a special alliance or coalition is formed. Cross-generational bonding, also referred to as emotional incest, is extremely harmful to children because they become caught in a confusing web of loyalty and deception. When a child is used to fulfill their mother's or father's disappointment and emptiness in the marital relationship, he or she loses the innocence of childhood. When the marriage is in crisis, the child takes on the responsibility for restoring family harmony because of his or her own need for self-preservation and survival. Cross-generational bonding is generally a symptom of severe family dysfunction (Bradshaw 23).

Getting a "Higher" Education

Indiana University is nestled in the wooded hills of Brown County in southern Indiana in a small town called Bloomington. Along with the outstanding school of music, excellent business program, and, of course, dental and medical schools, IU is more popularly known for its reputation as a party school, a well-deserved reputation!

Drugs were abundant on campus when I was there in the late seventies and early eighties. According to my niece, drugs were still easily obtained with a nominal amount of effort. Prescription drugs are sold for abuse equally with illicit street drugs. Today, lots of kids use Prozac, Xanax, Ritalin, Adderall, Oxycontin, and Vicodin in order to get high. Our local news has profiled students twice in the last month at the University of Texas who are using Adderall to study and binge drink. One female claimed to have faked ADHD symptoms to get a prescription. She now sells the extra pills to her sorority sisters during exams. Another male student proclaimed he felt like a genius on the drug and it enabled him to keep going after the hangovers he suffered from long party weekends. (This guy sounds like a genius to me!) Snorting these drugs like cocaine has become a popular way to pass the blood-brain barrier and intensify the buzz. More often than not, they are consumed simultaneously with alcohol.

I always had an innate fascination with and absolutely no fear of drugs. Back then, the dissolution of my parents' marriage left me depressed and confused. I started experimenting with a variety of substances that were going around campus. Hypnotics like prescription Placidyls and Quaaludes, or 714s as they were known, were a popular prescription drug of abuse back then. I had a friend that was known as "The Quaalude Dude" because of his Quaalude use. We had adorned our dorm rec room for his birthday party with big Quaalude tablet mobiles that hung from the ceiling as decoration. Kids often mixed Quaaludes and alcohol (a deadly combination) to further intensify their high. I liked the buzz from "ludes" but they left me feeling hungover, somewhat like alcohol.

Various dorm and frat parties would offer partiers a "window pane punch" in addition to the more traditional kegs of beer. Windowpane is LSD or blotter acid, as it is commonly known. Another friend from our dorm was affectionately called "Tripper" because of his frequent use of psychedelics. Psilocybin mushrooms and peyote were also available for the more naturally inclined experimenter. Speed in the form of black beauties, Christmas trees, and crystal kept students awake to study for final exams. Cocaine was around, but the average student did not have the budget for it. I personally hated the way it and speed made me feel. I was all jittery with diarrhea and an upset stomach. Plus, I couldn't stop talking, and it annoyed the crap out of people! Alcohol was the most commonly abused drug on campus. Weed and hashish were available everywhere and was made little issue of. Nearly everyone I knew smoked pot, and I found it preferable to the awful hangovers, drunken public displays, and the personal controversy that always seemed to erupt around alcohol consumption. Marijuana was so accepted back then. I remember a police officer asking me to put out a joint that my friends and I were smoking on the grounds of the Student Commons. "Why, of course, officer," I sheepishly replied. Can you imagine that happening now?

I quickly learned what drugs felt good and what drugs did not agree with my chemistry. Every time I used a stimulating drug, I regretted it. After a couple of harrowing experiences where I had to talk myself down for hours, I quickly adopted a pot-only policy. I would jokingly tell my friends I lived too close to the edge to do major drugs and I didn't want to end my days in a round room with padded walls, twisting my hair around my forefinger! How insightful that policy would turn out to be, and how relative that experience would later become in helping me to identify the adverse reaction I was having to a psychoactive drug. That's how I had known to get off the Zoloft. I had experienced a much milder version of this reaction in my previous experimental drug use. However, it had never occurred to me that an antidepressant was a *stimulant*. Duh!

I reveled in my days on the IU campus. Although I struggled to define myself and to learn to love and relate to others, I learned some very valuable life lessons there. Unfortunately, I would hurt several people that cared about me. Acting out my fear and confusion, I would look for love in all the wrong places, hoping someone could melt the icy cool of my intellect and touch the warmer, softer side of my spirit. It made me appear to be both promiscuous and capricious. I had very few loyalties to anyone else and was a waking nightmare for any young man who dared to try to love me. Little did anyone else know it was because I didn't trust anyone. Everyone I loved had hurt me. So, in turn, I built thick walls around my heart and my spirit in order to protect them. I certainly didn't love myself. That would not come until much later.

Married to my Best Friend

Rod, my life partner, husband, best friend, and the father of my son, and I have been together for twenty years now. Our marriage has definitely had its peaks and valleys. We were divorced in 1992 and remarried in 1994. We have weathered many storms together over the years. In spite of our many differences, we are very close at heart. Our relationship has provided the support and structure I've needed to remain as healthy as I have these past twelve years. It has been Rod's unconditional love and support that has salvaged our family and marriage in times when I have struggled with my family-of-origin dysfunction, disillusionment, health, moods, and addictions.

Rod and I met in 1984, shortly after we had both relocated to Texas. My first corporate job out of college was with the Indiana Medicaid Program for a Texas-based company, EDS (Electronic Data Systems). Back then, it was still owned by H. Ross Perot and had just been featured in a best-selling book by Ken Follet, *On the Wings of Eagles.* The book chronicled the story of a privately orchestrated rescue of American businessmen that were working for EDS and held hostage in Iran. Corporate spirit ran high. I was thrilled when, after only one year, I was promoted to the company's home base in Texas. Rod had just gotten out of the navy. He moved south from his native Wisconsin in order to escape the cold winters to which he had become unaccustomed while stationed in Hawaii. He decided to join his younger brother, Gary, who lived on the gulf coast in Corpus Christi.

Rod and I moved into the same apartment complex within weeks of one another. It was love at first sight (at least for me), and our romance was a whirlwind. We had only dated a month when I invited Rod to move in with me. We had been living together for three months when I proposed on Rod's birthday, which was also Sadie Hawkins Day. We met, dated, and were married in just nine months total.

It was six weeks before our wedding date when a superior who recognized my writing skills sent me on special assignment to EDS Government Services. I worked with a proposal writing team on the contract rebid for the Indiana Medicaid account. It was so exciting to be staying in the pulse of the nation's capital. EDS was located in Bethesda, Maryland, right outside of Washington, DC. I was able to make several trips into the capital during my six-week assignment.

Unfortunately, the rebid was not successful, and there was no job in Indiana for me to return to. That is how I ended up permanently relocating to Texas. I had moved to Corpus Christi to become a provider relations rep for the Texas Medicaid Program. My job was to call on doctors with our company's registered nurses concerning Medicaid billing problems and utilization review issues. On one of these visits, I met the McNeil Pharmaceutical rep while in an office waiting room. He was working with his district manager. That was my shoe in to the pharmaceutical industry. My previous political grooming and loyal corporate spirit from EDS served me well in the pharmaceutical industry. I enjoyed a prosperous, successful career and received multiple awards and numerous promotions.

After leaving McNeil, I later worked for Syntex Laboratories, Bristol-Myers Squibb, Abbott Laboratories, and Forest Laboratories. However, during my last three years spent with Abbott and Forest, I worked as an independent contractor on a part-time basis. This brought a completely different air and dynamic to the job. In the late 1990s, this cheaper form of contract labor would become the newest tool in the industry to increase voice share in the market and would seriously change the face and reputation of the detail rep. In 1994, there were estimated to be 35,000 full-time reps calling on physicians and detailing drugs. By 1998, that number exceeded 56,000, about one rep for every eleven doctors (Strand 48). Contract reps came from all areas of sales, were not nearly as well-trained, and had no incentive to self-educate. The quality of information the doctors were receiving began declining rapidly. Reps started piling up four and five deep in office waiting rooms as companies jockeyed for additional exposure in busy practices.

Rod continued supporting my career advancement for several years while he attended college. He lost credits at University of Houston when we relocated for my hospital job promotion. After I left McNeil, we also decided to leave Houston and moved back to Corpus Christi to have the baby. That allowed Rod to finish his degree at what is now Texas A&M in Corpus Christi. I went to work for a small, biotech firm called Syntex Laboratories and settled back into the sales territory I had worked initially. It was an immediate culture shock for me. Having recently worked with ultraconservative cultures in EDS and McNeil, to say the least, Syntex was extremely open and free-spirited in its corporate culture. I gawked in amazement at my first national sales meeting where professional women sported short leather skirts, bare legs, and open-toed shoes. Syntex was founded by the Stanford University researcher who discovered the birth control pill. The corporate culture reflected, not only the carefree, Bohemian attitudes of the California coast lifestyle, but those of the advent of the sexual revolution as well. Hijinks among sales reps and even management were continually rumored at meetings where wine and liquor flowed freely and reps had adjoining hotel rooms.

Rod finally obtained his bachelor's degree right before he was reactivated in the naval reserves and deployed to Desert Storm in 1991. Austin was eighteen months old at the time. Of course, the stress and fear surrounding Rod's absence caused my anxiety and insomnia to return. Unaware of my previous dependence on the drug, my doctor once again prescribed Xanax. The vicious cycle of addiction and withdrawal returned and continued.

11

God's Call to Loving Arms: A Spiritual Awakening

God's Call to Loving Arms

A gentle call awakened me in the middle of the night.
At first, I thought I dreamed it...but I heard a voice, all right!
I felt this strange familiarity—like meeting an old friend—
as this voice began to educate, explain, and comprehend
the things that I had gone through...the childhood pain I'd felt...
and with each soothing revelation the ice began to melt.
The feelings all came pouring out like rain, so soft and sweet,
and in the wake of all the cleansing tears that fell upon my sheets
was an aura of acceptance—almost humble gratitude—
for each and every lesson that life's heartaches had imbued.
For God had come to show me the strength that I had gained
and the countless other children who could profit from my pain.
The little girl who cried that night surrendered all that was
and drifted back to sleep assured his words would be her cause!
And though the voice had faded as I faced the morning's dawn,
the memory of its peaceful lilt continues lingering on.
Occasionally, it makes its way into my silent space
reminding me that I am still protected by his grace.
And every now and then, when my ego shows its pride
that voice of understanding comes to reassure—not chide!
It tells me he forgives me and extends his loving arms
and reminds me that illusions cannot do me any harm!
He gives me the security to err...to fail...to grow.
Since I heard God's call to loving arms,
I don't believe—I know!

Gwen Olsen (1994)

It is amazing how the pieces of the puzzle called life all come together in hindsight. Things appearing completely unrelated one to another are later revealed to have been intricately tied to an outcome or event. Such is the case with my childhood, family, education, career, advocacy, and other life experience.

Was it karma I would be the repeated victim of serious drug reactions? Probably, I cannot know for sure. I do know that each step of my life up to this point has lead to the writing of this book and the mission that has become the cornerstone of my existence since Meg died.

In fact, I was advised of and prepared for the writing of this book nearly a decade ago in the mystical experience I recount in my poem that serves as its subtitle. The poem came to me two weeks to the day and hour after I had my conversation with God. It was a confirmation that what I had experienced was real, not imagined or hallucinated as some might suggest.

God didn't speak to me in the throes of madness, but he came to me in the quiet of the night a couple of years after I had embarked on this spiritual journey. My ego had been completely debased, and I had opened my mind to infinite possibilities. It was then that I hit rock bottom emotionally and fell seemingly through to another level of consciousness, an abyss of knowledge, wisdom, compassion, and unconditional love of self. I had what is known in near-death experiences as a panoramic life review. I was allowed to see all of the events that had lead up to that point in my life in order to deliver me to that very meeting with God and the fulfillment of my special calling on this planet. I was reborn and my dis-ease of spirit was healed.

Do I believe this happened to me because of the mental illness? Partially…at least I believe the illness was a catalyst. However, my conversation with God was mostly the result of an angry cry I had made from the angst and pain at the depths of my soul, an exasperated plea for answers and an invocation to take over my life or give me the courage to end it. It states in the Bible, "Ask and it will be given to you; seek and you shall find. Knock and the door shall be opened to you" (Matthew 7:7). I had asked God questions that I yearned desperately to have him answer, and I had asked him to claim my life. He did both of these things. He just didn't do it at that exact moment in time because I was not yet prepared to receive his grace.

Psychospiritual Integration

As I mentioned earlier, I turned my back on conventional medicine and sought alternative therapies in order to heal. Although I know it was my own inner healer that delivered me from my mental torment and physical hell, I am extremely grateful to the wise, compassionate pioneers in psychotherapy who helped me access the healing power within. Those individuals embraced and applied the knowledge that psyche is the root word in psychology. Psyche means soul or spirit.

Perhaps it is a result of the brain damage I sustained, or maybe it is the product of the psychospiritual integration I have experienced through various therapeutic techniques, but I no longer remember all the nasty details of my entire childhood storyline. Some memories are certainly more poignantly painful than others, but most have been replaced by or attached to more pleasant healing experiences that I've had since in therapy. These therapeutic techniques actually diffused the negative feelings I had surrounding those memories.

It is difficult to describe or articulate the profound emotional and psychological healing I have experienced in some of the most unusual, if not controversial, new paradigm psychotherapeutic programs. However, my intellect does not need to comprehend a truth my heart, body, mind, and soul illustrate. I am grateful I was lead in this direction before it was too late for me. Before my own belief systems made my brain a bowl of oatmeal. Among the various techniques and therapies I have explored are chiropractic, yoga, aromatherapy, homeopathy, acupuncture, massage therapy, Ayurvedic medicine, herbal and nutritional supplementation, Reiki, transpersonal psychology, transformational breathwork, psychodrama, mask-making, trance dance, shadow work, mandala art, guided imagery, journaling, meditation, small group therapy, one-on-one life coaching, hypnosis, masterminding, visualization, and orthomolecular psychiatry.

The founder of Eupsychia, the psychospiritual recovery foundation that changed my life, Jacquelyn Small, said something to me I will never forget. "Often the only difference between a mystic and a psychotic is who they're talking to." How true that would prove to be in my experience. After you have been formally diagnosed as some form of *crazy*, everything you say or experience is suspected as delusional, a product of your mental illness.

For this reason, I have refrained from sharing the details of some of the most blissful, beautiful miracles of my life, except with my husband and closest loved ones, less someone lock me up and throw away the key! Even the folks I did tell listened with wide eyes and puzzled expressions as they tried to discern whether or not I was on solid ground. Here was the family's no-nonsense scientist speaking to them from previously unendorsed platforms of the etheric, spiritual side of human existence. Whatever they thought, they couldn't discount my obvious behavioral changes and newfound zeal for life.

I no longer carry the baggage of the anger that once consumed me because of all of the egregious transgressions made by the adults that destroyed my childhood innocence. I discovered that it required a massive amount of energy to retain the emotional charge and remember details surrounding those memories. Releasing them felt so freeing! At one time, forgiving someone signified defeat to me, an admission I was letting someone off the hook, so to speak. Now, I realize forgiveness is a tremendous spiritual gift and the key to freeing oneself from old wounds and fears. Forgiveness has renewed my emotional bond to my mother and father. Having accepted sole responsibility for my choices as an adult, I can now appreciate the tremendous spiritual strength I gained from having exercised those muscles early in life under their tutelage.

Learning to love myself has been an ongoing task. I can still be my own worst critic. Occasionally, I allow negative self-talk to filter in but, now, more likely than not, I catch it. It took embracing the wounded child I had been and forgiving her for being afraid, being calloused, running from those who hurt her, from judging herself so harshly, and for hurting herself and others. When I had finally dealt with the pain and dysfunction of my childhood, I was able to move forward as a healthier adult. I was prepared to take care of myself with fewer self-defeating habits and healthier relationship boundaries. I was better capable of being a parent to my son and an advocate for other children, as well as the protectorate and caretaker of my own inner child. Love truly does heal all wounds. Even self-love is a miraculous tonic!

I have accepted the fact I march to the tune of a different drummer. I think that has made me more tolerant of other people's differences. I seem to notice the things I have in common with others rather than the things that separate me from them. Maybe that is because I have felt excluded for the majority of my life. When I wasn't excluded, I felt like a fraud. I am at peace now with who I am as well as who I am not.

Someone once asked me, if I had it to do all over again, would I make the same choices? I didn't even hesitate before I responded, "Yes, I would." There was a good reason. The journey has been irreplaceable.

I saw a segment of *60 Minutes* about a young hiker, Aaron Ralston, who amputated his own arm in order to save his life in a hiking accident. It was a miraculous story of courage, faith, wisdom, and strength. This brave soul survived six days without food and three days without water. He lost forty-five pounds and twenty-five percent of his blood supply while he was trapped between a canyon wall and a boulder. He further had the presence of mind and inspiration to break two bones in his arm, amputate the arm with a dull pocket knife, tourniquet the wound, hike several miles, and rappel a 600-foot canyon wall in order to be rescued.

To me, the most remarkable thing Aaron said in his interview was, if he had it to do all over again, he would choose to have the experience he had in that canyon rather than not. The experience had molded him, rebirthed him into the human being he is now.

I understood exactly what he meant. As horrible as his ordeal was, he would choose to do it again because of the gifts of spirit he received for having overcome his obstacles with faith, prayer, inspiration, and ingenuity. As a result, life was much richer and fuller as well as appreciated by Aaron. He had been reborn in that dark night of the soul and would always have his so-called disability as a humbling reminder of the battle he had so bravely fought and won. It would serve as his trophy of triumph.

When we are faced with our own mortality, we can touch depths of the psyche that were unattainable before. We question all of our previous concepts and judgments for the basis of reality as we know it. We acquiesce to spirit, in other words, *surrender*, and ask for a miracle. The miracle then manifests as a by-product of the energetic shift in consciousness that had faith in a miraculous outcome.

"God's Call to Loving Arms" is a call to action, not war. In fact, as I write this, I am gently reminded that war is war, regardless of the cause. I try not to be as guilty of polluting the world with my own negative thought forms about the warmongers and sorcerers (be they in the White House or in the ivory towers of corporate America), as they are of polluting our minds and planet with their propaganda.

Sometimes the best way to make a difference is to be the difference. As Norman Vincent Peale said, "Change your thoughts and you change your world."

Shattered Lives, Broken Dreams, and Hell on Earth

As I look at the photographs, it is so sad. Four generations of women…the lost potential…the shattered dreams…the broken marriages…the drug and alcohol abuse…the wounded children. The repercussions just go on and on.

Some will say, "Well, this was bound to happen. It proves that mental illness is genetic." I can't help but wonder to what degree psychiatric drugs contributed to the breakdown of my family structure and its stability. I am even willing to say it was not the fault of the drugs, per se, although we all reacted negatively and had brain dysfunction following psychiatric therapy. However, I do think it is the fault of a society that thinks the dis-eases of the spirit can be solved as though they were medical issues and treated with drugs as solutions, the quick fix, pill-popping mentality the pharmaceutical companies propagate. I do blame a society whose ignorance makes mental illness carry such a heavy stigma. Not only do people suffer from the ravages of the damn illness itself, but they must also hide in shame for fear of discovery. I further feel indignant about the fact that bipolar illness is considered a serious disease, but those who live with it rarely have medical benefits comparable to other serious illness coverage. Society has consistently discriminated against those labeled as mentally ill. As a result, most people diagnosed as such have become outcasts of society (Whybrow 257). The loving support of family, friends, and the community is the only hope for a person who suffers from a mood disorder. Again, love heals all wounds of the spirit. Drugs are a Band-Aid at best!

Psychiatry leans too heavily on the prescription pad and ignores the root of the patient's problems by treating only the overt symptoms. Few relationships are formed with the modern-day psychiatrist. He generally monitors your medication progress in fifteen-minute appointments and leaves the talk therapy to the psychologists. I believe it is essential in healing to have what is referred to as a therapeutic alliance. There must be a mutual respect and trust in the relationship with your therapist. Hmmm, that means, if mental illness were disproved to be a biochemical imbalance of the brain, then most psychiatrists would be out of a job. That might explain why doctors are still doling out scripts for everyday emotional issues that need to be dealt with rather than sedated, huh?

Any of the brave scholars who currently dare to speak out and challenge the ethics of biopsychiatry are quickly discredited by their peers, and their reputation is bashed in the scientific community. Psychiatrists are, after all, in competition with psychologists who cannot prescribe drugs. To have one of their own suggest there may be more humane treatments than drug restraint is not only insulting to their training, but it is also a threat to their economic security!

You cannot medicate away the dis-ease of a disquieted spirit. Depression and other forms of mental illness can be tremendous catalysts for spiritual transformation, just like other life-threatening illness or trauma. Remember the old joke about the patient who tells the doctor, "Doc, it hurts when I do this…" and the doctor replies, "Well, then don't do that!" There is a ton of practical advice in that joke. Depression is a form of mental pain. If we take away our ability to feel that pain by medicating ourselves into states of euphoria and/or catatonia, then we are not able to intellectually discern what not to do that is hurting us! It is necessary to feel our experience and integrate it into our awareness in order to have good mental health. It is experiencing our feelings that make us vital human beings. If we do not turn off our hectic outer realities occasionally and get in touch with our inner being, we miss valuable opportunities for self-renewal and growth. If we never get to the root of what actually hurts, how can we ever hope to fix it? Depression can be the spirit's way of demanding physical rest, emotional introspection, and spiritual change. It is an invitation to explore what you are doing that hurts you and to stop doing it.

In my own experience, I have found fear to be the most destructive, malignant contributor to my mental and emotional disease. It may be human nature to be greedy, self-righteous, self-serving, and fearful of other men, but that is not our spiritual nature. When life's experiences teach us as children to be guarded, secretive, suspicious, and afraid of our fellow man, then we set ourselves up to attract to us our greatest fears in life. It is a metaphysical principle. Whatever we put great mental and emotional energy into, we manifest into our reality. What we expect, we get. Caught in the boomerang of our own dismay and disillusion as children, we can begin a downward spiral early in life that dictates the bulk of our adult experience later on. Any internal chaos that goes unchecked will eventually wreak havoc in one's outer reality. Even the sharpest, most brilliant mind is at risk if it occupies space with destructive emotions. You can create your own nightmares, or you can manifest your dreams. It is up to you. Heaven is a state of mind and can be lived here on earth if you so choose…but then, so can hell.

Maintaining Healthy Boundaries in Relationships

The truth is, no matter how much you love someone, it is sometimes necessary to end toxic relationships. You know a relationship is toxic to you when the other person rarely contributes anything positive to your life or mental well-being. When you are around that person, you feel uncomfortable, anxious, or depressed because they emit a negative energy or are otherwise self-absorbed or self-destructive. If you find yourself involved in the drama of someone else's life to the extent that it negatively impacts you and your immediate family, then that is a toxic relationship! People who trigger our own issues are often attracted to us in order to teach us valuable lessons. Usually, part of that lesson is learning to set healthy boundaries with others that may not be good for us or learning to lovingly let go of those relationships. It is impossible to help someone who will not help themselves, and wisdom cannot be taught. However, it is entirely too easy to fall into the trap of viewing the world from the negative perspective of someone else, thereby subjecting ourselves to the same pitfalls in life they are creating.

Emotional Cutoff

In psychological terms, withdrawing from relationships with loved ones without resolution is referred to as emotional cutoff. Dealing with emotional cutoff in family relationships can be very painful. Family members generally utilize this strategy when they are unable to resolve serious conflict. The people involved normally care a lot about one another, but they do not know how to constructively deal with that love (Bradshaw 69).

Over the years, when I have felt violated to the point of no return, I have severed a number of close relationships. As a child, I feared reprisal or isolation if I expressed my anger. So, because of that, I learned to shove my anger down inside and redirect it toward myself. When I was exceptionally angry, I would separate myself from the person I was angry with, often never reestablishing contact. In spite of all the years of therapy and healing work and after having read more than 150 self-help, theology, and psychology books, I still withdraw from emotional conflict in relationships. This is also a learned behavior. The emotional cutoff appears to increase in intensity with each generation in my family, which makes our history both strange and secretive.

I don't pretend this behavior makes me any healthier than any other family member. In fact, the opposite is true. I know intellectually that the person who runs from their family-of-origin is as emotionally dependent as the one who never leaves home. To this end, I am continually trying to establish boundaries in all of my relationships that do not threaten my health or emotional well-being. Those attempts are frequently met with contempt by family members who wish to keep me enmeshed in our dysfunctional family dynamics.

12

Birth of a Child Advocate

"I slept and dreamt that life was joy.
I awoke and saw that life was service.
I acted and, behold, service was joy."

—Tagore

The buyout and merger frenzy of the early 1990s finally caught up to me in 1994 when Roche Laboratories purchased Syntex. I had just completed five years of tenure and gotten vested with Syntex, having survived two previous corporate downsizings. In 1991, I had been promoted to a specialty rep. In 1993, I had been awarded district rep of the year for the ob-gyn sales team. I was also invited that year to interview for a lobbyist position. (I didn't get it, thank God!) Just three weeks before Christmas, I got my walking papers from Roche via Fed Ex. After all my hard work, I was stunned! My whole identity had been wrapped up in being the "Syntex rep." I had no idea what I would do next. Fortunately, this would turn out to be a huge blessing in disguise. My severance package provided me with a full year's salary, and I was eligible for unemployment benefits as well. That allowed me the luxury of taking time off to do some intensive healing work and to redirect my focus and energy into helping others. That's when I heard about Court Appointed Special Advocates (CASA).

Frankly, I never really cared much for kids when I was one. I was an only child for six years before my sister was born. It was difficult for me to identify with other children because I had to grow up so quickly in order to survive.

But, armed with the firsthand experience of how family dysfunction can harm a child, I decided to make a difference for someone else. I volunteered and was trained to be a CASA for the Travis County court system. A CASA volunteer is assigned to abused and neglected children removed from their parents and caught in the state's foster care system. The CASA serves as the child's voice in court advocating for the child's best interests and follows the child's case through the system until its completion.

At the final disposition, sometimes I, as the child's CASA, would be the only remaining constant in the child's case after a parade of welfare caseworkers, student attorney-ad-litems, and foster families traipsed through their lives. The system was inept and cumbersome, frustrating me to the hilt at times!

My choice to be a CASA was a special calling and was some of the most excruciating, yet rewarding, work I have ever done. The rewards of the heart are so much greater than those of the ego. Even in the midst of such despair, one feels heady from the joy of giving in this way. I advocated as a CASA for five years. During that time, I helped seven children find safe, permanent homes.

The most amazing thing about the service work I have done is how therapeutic it has been personally. As you reach out to help others and shift your focus from your wants, needs, and problems to those of the less fortunate, it has a remarkable healing effect on everyone involved. I literally felt embarrassed I had ever considered myself an abuse victim. The children I worked with had suffered unspeakable neglect, abuse, and abandonment. Sometimes, we must get knee-deep in the muck of human catastrophe in order to learn life's most valuable lessons. It is true that light shines its brightest in the darkest places.

As a CASA, part of my responsibility was to follow up on the progress of parents and the recommended treatments ordered by the court in the Child Protective Services (CPS) service plan. Alarmingly, I began noticing rampant use of psychiatric drugs with children in the system. Children as young as three and four years of age were readily given antidepressants, antipsychotics, and stimulants such as Ritalin and Adderall.

In one case I was assigned with five little children (four boys and one girl ages infant to seven years), all except the baby boy and the little girl were taking major psychiatric drugs. These boys struggled daily with their foster families and teachers drugging them to subdue their emotional outbursts. During our visits, sometimes they would fall asleep upright in their chairs. Other times, they would run about the room wildly out of control, screaming, kicking, biting, and cursing at their mother or caseworker.

I will never forget the first time I saw the children, particularly the oldest boy, who was then five years old. I had arrived in the CPS parking lot for a meeting with the children's mother after their visit. When I pulled up, this little boy was screaming and flailing his arms as the caseworker attempted to stuff him and his siblings into the back seat of her car. He managed to escape, rolled down the window, and then bellowed at his mother, "Fucking bitch!" as she retreated into the building. Suddenly, both of his little hands flew straight into the air, extending their middle fingers. I was flabbergasted!

After reading the extensive case history on this family, I learned the children's parents had also been in the system and were themselves the products of abusive, neglectful environments. They had met in a juvenile detention center. The father was a gangbanger that had been habitually in and out of prison. Both parents had issues with alcohol and illegal substance abuse. The mother had been diagnosed with a borderline personality disorder and ordered to take Prozac by the court psychiatrist.

For two years, a picture of the oldest boy (age four at the time of the photo) adorned my desk as a reminder why I had become a CASA. There was a purplish bruise from the imprint of a cowboy boot heel that covered the entire left side of his face. It was a gift from his drunken father for intervening in a fight between his parents! This little boy had become the self-appointed protectorate of his mother and younger siblings at a very early age. It certainly explained to me why he was outraged with his mother for having abandoned him.

I would face a number of my own demons working with these children. Their mother would vacillate between docile and explosive moods in my presence, which sent me reeling emotionally. The father would beat the mother during drunken rages, only to have her take him back...again and again. The children were utterly helpless at the hands of their doctors and caretakers, and they were forced to take drugs that were obviously restraining rather than helping them. It all distressed me greatly. I tried to get the court to listen, but who was *I* to challenge the psychiatrist's recommendations? These were very angry, deeply disturbed children that required medication in order to function at home and in school. Yes, they were deeply disturbed indeed, but they were also three-, four-, and five-year-old little boys that needed to feel loved and secure, not drugged and betrayed! They were not even old enough to understand, let alone verbalize, what the drugs they took were doing to them. Of course they were angry. I was angry, too!

The following excerpts from my case notes recorded during interviews with foster parents, teachers, and therapists of the children support my concerns and chronicle the progression and magnitude of this problem over time. The names of the children have been changed in order to protect their identities.

8/18—Spoke with children's new foster mother. She said Juan Carlos was prescribed clonidine following his psychiatric evaluation. (Dr. Numnuts works for the placement agency.) She said he was adjusting to the medication, but initially was very lethargic on the drug. [It should be noted that clonidine is an alpha-antagonist also known as Catapres. It is indicated to treat high blood pressure and is not approved for use in children under the age of eighteen. However, psychiatrists frequently prescribe it for children with attention deficit/hyperactivity disorder.]

9/4—Spoke with foster parents. Juan Carlos appears to be responding to his medication but is having behavioral difficulties off and on. They say, Roberto, the four year old, has gotten more difficult to handle and they are going to talk to the doctor about getting him on medication as well.

9/12—Spoke with foster father. He said the boys had been acting-out considerably and that the youngest boy, Albert, age 2, was using the 'F' word frequently of late. He said he's been very aggressive and kicks a lot. Foster father emphatically remarked that he didn't think Juan Carlos' dose of .1 mg. of clonidine twice a day was working.

10/30—Supervised visit between mother and children. Talked briefly with foster parents who said Juan Carlos is doing better now that his medication has been increased (remember to check on this). Mother basically ignored the children as she tried to catch me up on the saga with their father. The baby is walking now and was all over the place as she explored her surroundings. There appears to be very little emotional bond between Mom and her baby. The kids started to get wild and restless, and Roberto started to hit, bite, kick, and talk back, which required him to be put in 'time-out.' This was the second occasion mother has appeared to have been up all night without having slept prior to the visit. When I questioned this, she said she had stopped taking her Prozac because the prescription ran out, and she was having difficulties sleeping. (Note: Mother's psych eval indicates passive aggressive tendencies and borderline personality traits.)

11/28—Placement Progress Meeting was held. Therapist say Juan Carlos is improving although he still has anger issues, and fights and takes things from other children. Juan Carlos doesn't respond well to punishment and starts bawling in time-out. Psychiatrist added imipramine to Juan Carlos' meds for bed-wetting issues but he is still wetting his pull-up diaper nightly. [Imipramine, also known as Tofranil, is a tricyclic antidepressant and is not approved for use in children under eighteen. Several deaths have been associated with the use of its main metabolite desipramine.]

Roberto—Has appointment with psychologist to check out the possibility of Fetal Alcohol Syndrome or neurological damage. Roberto is very absent-minded and has outbursts of aggression and anger. Foster father says he doesn't listen well, but hasn't been put on medication yet.

Albert—Now 2 ½, is developmentally on target and always smiling. He has started to finally make eye contact with adults. He is not currently in therapy or on any meds.

Maria—Now 17 months, walking, and very content to play alone, is developmentally on target.

5/28—Children were returned to their mother. Juan Carlos has about one month's supply of his medication according to the foster mother.

6/15—Judge Hathaway removed the kids again today and they were placed back with the foster family. It was discovered that the father—who had been forbidden visitation without services—had been with the children every week since they'd gone back home. Not only that, but mother had left the children in state-funded daycare for the two weeks they were with her and she was unemployed! Mother went berserk in court. Next hearing is in six weeks.

6/19—Contacted foster parents. They say Roberto is taking it the hardest and is very angry. Juan Carlos' bed-wetting continued and encopresis has gotten worse—he was having frequent involuntary bowel movements. Discovered today that parents of the children had gotten married on April 12, because mother is pregnant again!

8/14—Children are not doing well at all according to their therapist and foster parents. They are all extremely aggressive and defiant. Juan Carlos started first grade on Tuesday and the younger boys are going to Head Start next week. Therapist is requesting Juan Carlos' meds be adjusted.

8/18—Attended Placement Progress Meeting. Juan Carlos' clonidine has been increased to .1 tablet three times daily, Wellbutrin has been added for depression. (Find out if imipramine was discontinued!) He has started wearing pull-ups again for bed-wetting and day-time encopresis. After return to foster family, his anger has increased as well as his aggressive behavior with siblings. His teacher called to report to foster parents that he is falling behind quickly in his studies, staring into space, not able to follow well in class. [It should be noted that Wellbutrin is an antidepressant not approved for use in children under eighteen.]

Roberto—Yesterday was his first day at Head Start. His aggression has been so serious he was given an EEG to rule out silent seizures. Nothing was found. Roberto is now wearing pull-ups at night for bed-wetting too. He is in play therapy with other children. An appointment with the psychiatrist is scheduled for next Monday.

Albert—Doesn't wet the bed like the older boys, but his behavior deteriorated over the past four months. He also has an appointment with the psychiatrist next Monday.

Maria—She had no special needs at this time but has become more aggressive in her own defense.

9/9—Talked with foster father who says kids are regressing horribly. Juan Carlos is falling behind at school. His teacher says he ignores her and won't respond to questions, and doesn't recognize words. Psychiatrist put Roberto on 5 mg. of Paxil but it doesn't seem to be doing any good. Albert was given 5 mg. of Adderall at his last psych evaluation. [It should be noted that Paxil is an SSRI antidepressant and Adderall is a combination of amphetamine and dextroamphetamine. Neither drug is approved for use in children under the age of eighteen, but both are frequently prescribed to children.]

9/12—Talked with foster mother following a teacher/parent conference for Juan Carlos. She said the teacher remarked that Juan Carlos appears to be 'jumpy and jittery.' Teacher said they were considering putting him in kindergarten because he couldn't answer even the simplest questions about letters. She also told me that Roberto and Albert are having difficulties at Head Start and have been sent home for aggressive behaviors repeatedly. They appear to be getting wilder rather than better on their drugs.

9/19—Spoke with Juan Carlos' teacher, who said that J.C. is there physically but not mentally. He won't do his homework. She's been giving him special assignments out of kindergarten books. She said she thinks he may be brain damaged—he doesn't respond when questioned, has inappropriate affect and a 'lost look' in his eyes.

9/30—Talked with caseworker who said the doctor had added 5 mg. of Adderall to Roberto's Paxil. She reported his aggression was out of control, and they had started him in another elementary school for early childhood. Head Start will no longer take him! Juan Carlos has improved somewhat since they lowered the dose of his clonidine again to twice daily. They also switched his antidepressant to Paxil. His teacher was complaining he appeared excessively drowsy in the afternoon.

10/12—Children's caseworker called to relate the following incident which occurred with the transporter yesterday. Apparently, following the visit with their mother, the children had to be corralled from the street. Then, while in transit, they attacked the transporter! Roberto pulled the emergency brake as they were driving at about 60 mph. Juan Carlos reportedly told Roberto to 'poke her eyes out and cut her titties off!' and began to spit, hit and bite her while she was driving. The caseworker was so traumatized that she refuses to transport the children any more. As a result, the caseworker said Juan Carlos has been switched from clonidine to Adderall and Paxil. Roberto's and

Albert's Adderall have been increased to 10 mg. daily. I asked about the combination use of Adderall with Paxil, she said the psychiatrist claimed they work better in combination." (Note: Could this incident have been caused by the children's meds?)

The children's progress continued to deteriorate. In December, the unborn baby boy arrived and was attached to the case. Parental rights were eventually terminated. Four of the children were placed in another state. The baby was put in a separate family, but all of them were placed for permanent adoption. They had lingered and suffered at the hands of the system for more than two years. This was the last case I would handle as a CASA. I had lost my faith in and respect for a system run amuck. The child welfare system had more problems than I was able to cope with. Plus, I just knew this was the end of that particular journey for me. Somehow, I knew it had fulfilled its purpose, so I walked away.

A Plea for the Children

Children are so vulnerable because of their smaller size, limited cognitive skills, and dependence on others. They are three times more likely to experience adverse drug reactions than adults. It is sad to think that state agencies responsible for child welfare would further exploit and abuse children in their custody by excessive use of psychiatric medications.

However, it is well known in the pharmaceutical industry that children are a lucrative market for drugs and are possibly the single most promising growth area in the industry. The mere fact that children are forced by parents and teachers to take medication ensures a compliant patient. That means refilled prescriptions and more sales. Psychiatric drugs are marketed aggressively for use in children. Antidepressant use is up, especially among kids age five and younger. According to Express Scripts data, antidepressant use in these kids doubled from 1998 to 2002, up one hundred percent (DeNoon). Eli Lilly even proposed a peppermint-flavored Prozac to market for children. (The FDA denied its application.) However, adolescents between the ages of twelve and seventeen are the biggest child consumers of antidepressants (Huffington).

Children have an increased risk for antidepressant-induced mania. In one clinical trial involving Prozac for depressed children, six percent were forced to drop out because of Prozac-induced mania—six percent! Internal documents for the FDA show a rate for mania of slightly above one percent. However, in the data submitted by the manufacturer for Prozac's approval, hypomania/mania was listed to occur at 0.7 percent (Breggin and Cohen 61). Quite the discrepancy, don't you think? But, remember, the approval trials were conducted on select adult candidates with mild to moderate depression. All serious psychiatric illness had been screened out. Therefore, one would expect these figures to increase in routine clinical practice because the average child who receives a prescription for an antidepressant is not screened for a potential predisposition to mania.

If you are a parent trying to determine if psychiatric medications are appropriate for your child, remember one thing: Most of these drugs have not been tested on and are, therefore, not approved to be used in children under the age of eighteen. Many may escalate your child's emotional issues. Children require love, attention, nurturing, and healthy boundaries to feel emotionally secure and well-adjusted. Even if the drugs manage to restrain or numb their feelings and behavior, if the root of their origin is not addressed, they will soon return, often with a vengeance, once the drugs are removed.

Developing brains are far more vulnerable to brain damage than adult brains. Damage received in childhood may only become apparent after the brain is fully developed. The drastic increases in cortisol produced by the SSRIs and SNRIs can cause brain damage. In addition, they can cause a multitude of serious physical reactions in children, such as impairment of linear growth and the interference with development and regeneration of liver tissue, kidneys, and muscles, and so forth (Tracy 2001). Most recently, Eli Lilly's new drug, Strattera, which was launched in 2002 and enjoyed $667 million in annual sales in 2004, received a bolded warning regarding the potential for severe liver injury. Strattera is a SNRI (the same category as Zoloft) and is indicated for attention deficit/hyperactivity disorder (ADHD) (Swiatek).

Stimulants such as Ritalin (methylphenidate) and Adderall (d-amphetamine and amphetamine mixture) can cause excessive stimulation of the brain and result in insomnia, seizure, agitation, irritability, nervousness, confusion and disorientation, personality changes, apathy, social isolation, sadness, and depression. They may also cause paranoia resulting in violence toward others.

Regulators removed Adderall XR from the Canadian market on February 9, 2005, because of reports linking the drug to twenty sudden deaths (fourteen children and six adults) and a dozen strokes, including two in children. (I wonder what our genius interviewed at UT would think about that?) The FDA evaluated these same reports and determined it did not feel the data warranted such action in the United States. Currently, there are approximately 700,000 Americans taking Adderall XR. Another 300,000 take Adderall. However, the FDA has modified Adderall use instructions to include a warning against use in patients with cardiovascular disease (Gardner, A.).

Furthermore, millions of children now taking Ritalin and Adderall in order to function better in school are being forced to do so for the benefit of the teaching institution or teacher, not the child! Many schools are ill-equipped to handle the needs of energetic children who have difficulty sitting quietly still for hours on end in overcrowded classrooms. These stimulants are used to promote compliance, obedience, reduced initiative, and reduced autonomy, making children in group settings easier to manage (Breggin and Cohen 66).

Even if your child has been diagnosed with ADHD, you need to be objective about your school's policy and determine if it has low tolerance for rambunctious kids. I would strongly suggest you explore other options before allowing your child to be subjected to the risks of psychiatric medications. With the proper dietary adjustments and the nutritional supplementation of Omega-3 essential fatty acids (EFAs), many symptoms of ADHD can be completely eradicated. If you are looking for a magic bullet in psychiatric medications, especially where children are concerned, you are playing *Russian roulette.*

Just in case you think I'm being an alarmist with that statement, consider this last tidbit about another ADHD drug that I found while browsing the FDA's Web site. It was also potentially prescribed to children. On February 10, 2005, the FDA and Alliant Pharmaceutical notified all health care professionals and consumers on their Web site about the recall of all Methilyn CT (methylphenidate HCL) 2.5, 5, and 10 milligram tablets. Their posting stated that some tablets may contain up to three times the active ingredient and could pose serious risk to some patients (U.S. Food 2005b). (Don't you think children might be the most vulnerable to this potential overdose?)

The Fine Line Crossed Between Legal and Illegal Drug Use

Our blatant hypocrisy where psychoactive drug use is concerned has not escaped the notice of our teenagers. These kids have grown up on Ritalin and other psychoactive substances prescribed by their doctors and endorsed by their parents. Meanwhile, their peers, as well as some parents, were abusing their prescription drugs and others in order to get high. The government has waged an open war on illicit drugs like marijuana and cocaine for years. Yet, we also need to aggressively teach our youth about the inherent dangers of prescription drug use so they don't have a false sense of security when they experiment just because something is legal and prescribed by a doctor. It isn't difficult to see why many kids feel society talks out of both sides of its mouth where drug use is concerned. For the most part, they have seen more of their friends die on prescription drugs than they have illicit ones.

For example, I have a half-brother, Ben, from my father's second marriage. (His mother, ironically, is the daughter of my dad's former mistress that I mentioned earlier.) He lives in Las Vegas. Ben is by passion, if not profession, a phenomenal rapper. His crew is called *Tha List.* Unfortunately, in his social circles, he started experimenting with drugs and alcohol very early (about the sixth grade). This earned him the nickname "Benzo," short for benzodiazepine. Ben became an alcoholic quickly and dropped out of school. Eventually, because of his drinking and drugging, he ended up on the wrong side of the law. Now Ben is twenty-two.

When we talked following Meg's death, my brother told me about two of his homies that had also recently died. One was killed in a car wreck (driving while intoxicated), and the other had died of an overdose of Xanax, methadone, and alcohol. Apparently, the last guy had actually died on the couch in Ben's apartment. Ben's comment to me was, "Wow, and now this thing with Megan. I feel like God has been throwing lightning bolts at my feet and all around me lately, trying to tell me something." Of course, my reply was, "Well, Ben, if you feel that way, maybe there's something to it!"

PARENT'S CREED
Author Unknown

If a child lives with criticism,
    He learns to condemn.

If a child lives with hostility,
    He learns to fight.

If a child lives with ridicule,
    He learns to be shy.

If a child lives with shame
    He learns to feel guilty.

If a child lives with tolerance,
    He learns to be patient.

If a child lives with encouragement,
    He learns confidence.

If a child lives with praise,
    He learns to appreciate.

If a child lives with security,
    He learns to have faith.

If a child lives with approval,
    He learns to like himself.

If a child lives with acceptance
    and friendship,

He learns to find love in the world.

13

A Betrayal of the Public Trust

"The world is a dangerous place, not because of those who do evil, but because of those who look on and do nothing."

—Albert Einstein

It is no small coincidence that, before I could even complete or publish this book, the press started reporting on the outrageous conflicts of interest existing between the FDA and the pharmaceutical industry. In recent months, several inside whistle-blowers from the FDA have come forward, exposing the intimidation of investigators who try to alert the public to potential risks affiliated with new drugs. Dr. David Graham, a twenty-year veteran investigator with the FDA, is one such champion. Dr. Graham questions the viability of a regulatory agency funded largely by the industry it regulates and has called the attention of Congress to several new drugs he considers to be potential time bombs.

Most people would be surprised to learn of the close financial ties between the FDA and the pharmaceutical industry. Thanks to the Prescription Drug User Fee Act of 1992, Congress allowed the FDA to collect user's fees from the pharmaceutical companies to help fund the approval of new drugs. This fee is up to $300,000 for each new drug application.

Before 1992, the FDA had a fairly unfriendly reputation in the industry as being too strict and bogged down by bureaucracy. However, since the introduction of the user's fees, the FDA has approved an unprecedented number of new drug applications in record speed. In fact, Total Approval Times, the time from the initial submission of a New Drug Application to the issuance of an Approval Letter, was cut from an average of twenty-three months to twelve months. Fast-tracking of priority applications was also cut in half, reduced from an average of twelve months to six months (Strand 36).

This appeared to be the perfect solution for the government. Pressure was mounting from special interest groups such as AIDS and cancer patients, who needed to acquire new drugs, and whose growing numbers startled Americans. It cannot be denied that the accelerated approval process may have saved the lives of thousands of patients desperately in need of these new drugs (Strand 41–42). However, the end result has been that a large number of dangerous chemicals, which in essence were "me too" drugs and provided no major advantages over existing therapies, have been unleashed on an unsuspecting American public without adequate testing and scientific data.

In the FDA approval process, a drug can fail numerous times in clinical trials to show efficacy (to be effective) and still be approved, as long as two or more studies show a statistical superiority over placebo. Drug companies carefully select patients and researchers to improve the probable outcomes of their trials (Breggin, *Talking Back to Prozac*, 47).

Remember, less than fifty percent of the serious adverse reactions to a new drug are identified by the FDA before its release on the market. The FDA relies largely on post-marketing surveillance to identify all of a new drug's adverse reactions. Even then, the FDA estimates only one to ten percent of all adverse reactions are reported. Only sixty-five full-time employees work at the FDA's office of Post-Marketing Drug Risk Assessment, and they monitor the 8,000 plus drugs that are currently on the market. Conversely, more than 1,400 employees staff the approval of new drugs (Strand 74). The result is that the American population has become the largest Phase IV clinical trial population on the planet. The ramifications of this imbalance will not be known in its entirety for some time yet to come.

This gross betrayal of the public trust undermines more than the health of select individuals. It subterfuges the entire health care system and diminishes one's belief/faith in his or her doctor and the remedies prescribed to heal him or her. If a patient is skeptical to begin with about the doctor's knowledge and/or motivations or is concerned about the safety of a drug prescribed, then healing is more elusive. After all, the gold standard, placebo comparison in clinical trials exists because the body and mind can heal themselves. This is an accepted fact among medical professionals. There is simply no other way to explain the miraculous recoveries and remissions that occur in some people with the mere suggestion they are receiving treatment. Inactive placebos are sugar pills…nothing more.

(It should be noted that Phase IV clinical trials are largely conducted for marketing purposes as well. For Phase IV trials, the doctors, rather than the patients, are carefully selected by the pharmaceutical manufacturer. Companies want influential doctors to get immediate exposure to their new drugs, so they pay doctors to enroll patients in their practices into Phase IV trials. The incentive paid is usually several hundred dollars per patient. You can see how a monetary incentive like that might sway a doctor to use a new drug rather than an older one for his patient. Quite frankly, the results of these Phase IV trials are rarely conducted under strict clinical guidelines, and most are never reported to the FDA) (Goozner 230, 238).

Follow the Leader

In all of my years working with doctors, I have never met one whom I felt would do intentional harm to a patient. Prescribing habits among physicians are varied (and believe me, poor prescribing is common), but this can be attributed to the fact that doctors receive little, if any, unbiased training about drugs following their residency. Nearly every educational opportunity or event they attend thereafter is funded or provided by the pharmaceutical industry.

Continuing Medical Education (CME) is a huge commercial enterprise. Currently, the Accreditation Council for Continuing Education accredits more than 100 for-profit companies. Medical education service suppliers receive nearly three-quarters of their income from pharmaceutical companies. These companies provide CME formerly available only in academic medical centers and medical schools. The rapid advance of medicine in recent years has forced large numbers of practicing physicians back into the classroom in order to keep up with the times (Kassirer 16).

Pharmaceutical companies eagerly support CME for the marketing opportunities they provide. In 2003, drug companies spent more than $1,500 per year on CME for each doctor in the United States. Their contributions represented seventy percent of all continuing education for doctors (Abramson 119). The CME companies are very savvy and know exactly what it takes to change a practicing physician's prescribing habits—deference to the recognized experts. In other words, doctors follow their leaders.

Medical education suppliers hire professional experts from either medical academic settings or community thought leaders, also referred to as key opinion leaders (KOLs). It is widely acknowledged that most of the top medical authorities in this country—and virtually all of the top speakers on medical topics—are employed in some capacity by one or more of the country's pharmaceutical companies (Kassirer 15–19). This is particularly true in the incestuous world of biopsychiatry.

As the press caught wind of the outlandish marketing excesses employed by the pharmaceutical industry in the late 1990s, CME became an even more important marketing tool. All of a sudden, for expense purposes, huge entertainment budgets were now shifting into continuing education. The excesses did not stop. They were just accounted for differently, that is, politically correctly. In 2002, under increasing public scrutiny, Pharmaceutical Research and Manufacturers of America (PhRMA) voluntarily imposed guidelines for permissible, modest offerings. These guidelines are poorly adhered to.

In addition to CME courses, doctors routinely attend medical conferences and other meetings in which pharmaceutical companies sponsor the affiliated symposia. Drug companies pay handsomely to have elaborate displays of their products at these meetings. Doctors meander through the display halls during their breaks, visiting with reps and stuffing large bags full of promotional trinkets and other goodies. It never ceased to amaze me how greedy some of these doctors could be. A particular example that comes to mind was a popular social event that was provided to doctors at medical conferences for years by one of my former employers, Syntex Laboratories. It was called "All Things Chocolate."

"All Things Chocolate" was by invitation only and consisted of a banquet hall full of the most decadent chocolate desserts and treats imaginable. Everything—chocolate mousse, cookies, ice cream, cheesecakes, and giant, chocolate candy sculptures—was served on dozens of help yourself banquet tables.

As a specialty rep, I was often requested to work conventions and medical conferences. I had been warned about the chaos that "All Things Chocolate" had provoked in the past. My colleagues referenced the event as a feeding frenzy, and I soon found out why.

Doctors and their wives would do anything to sneak into this event, telling elaborate stories to doormen about their lost invitations. Once inside, women would literally open their handbags and scoop handfuls of expensive chocolates and other treats off the tables into them. I witnessed one Indian woman who opened her sari, fashioning it to serve as a tote. With one fell-swoop of her forearm, she took a complete display of Godiva chocolates. Her husband stood by nervously, acting as though he hadn't seen her. It was outrageous!

On the local level, sales reps also provide funding for journal clubs, staff meetings, grand rounds, and other educational opportunities in hospitals. The rep generally brings food and is given an opportunity to display and promote his or her products in return. There is always a quid pro quo expected in this industry, which, in essence, translates to "you do something for me, and I do something for you."

Several doctors in private practice take advantage of these relationships by requiring reps to see them by appointment only over lunch. This policy routinely provides food and drinks for their staff. Toward the end of my career, I started to exclusively use a catering service because of the sheer number of appointments that required meals to be carried in. Many offices offer both breakfast as well as lunch appointments. I once saw a local employment ad that listed "meals provided by pharmaceutical reps" as a benefit for a medical receptionist position. The competition among different reps is not limited to their drugs either. It would irk me something fierce when office personnel would pit me against other sales reps by saying, "so-and-so brought Olive Garden last week…" in order to drop the name of a major competitor. As a cardiology specialist, I often spent $200+ for a luncheon that might provide me a two-minute opportunity to talk with the doctor…if I was lucky!

"Shadowing" the Opinion Leaders

The sun was just starting to rise as I raced through the parking garage into the hospital operating room (OR). The previous day, I had accompanied one of my cardiologists in the cath lab (where many cardiac procedures are performed) of the same hospital to "shadow" him and learn about the various procedures. This was a popular way for reps to win time and establish rapport with influential specialists that might not see pharmaceutical reps otherwise. For the mere cost of an anatomical heart model ($400), a cardiologist would allow me to spend a half-day or so observing him interact with patients. A cardiovascular surgeon, who was known by all the female reps for his machismo, had stuck his head in to provoke my instructing cardiologist and invited me to come and see a "real doctor at work." He had given me instructions to meet him the next morning in the OR for an aortic valve replacement.

I was a little apprehensive about how I would handle the whole thing. I don't have a very strong stomach and have never been able to tolerate even the sight of my own blood without fainting. However, my numerous years of "surgery over lunch" with graphic films depicting bloody procedures had desensitized me somewhat to the blood of others.

The surgical team and anesthesiologist arrived before the surgeon and began prepping the patient for surgery. The elderly woman having the procedure looked frail and frightened as they prepared her for anesthesia. The nurses spoke reassuringly as they inserted her IV line. I was instructed to take my place behind the patient drape with the anesthesiologist, and I was given a stool to stand on so that I could overlook the patient's chest cavity. As soon as the patient was under, I was struck by the marked change in demeanor among the surgical team. They started laughing and making crude remarks about the old woman's mastectomy and other physical traits. Under the circumstances, it seemed irreverent. I was grateful when the surgeon finally arrived and the nurses, all in a flutter, broke off their antics.

This was a fascinating educational experience. It was unlike any I have had since. I watched in awe and amazement as the chest of this eighty-four-year-old woman was cut open with a saw and her ribs were pried apart with a spreader in order to access her heart. I stood mesmerized in that position for nearly five hours, just observing this medical miracle.

The surgeon removed material from the woman's aorta that resembled tooth enamel. I heard it clunk as he dropped it onto the instrument tray for me to view. The doctor openly flirted with me as the hours of the procedure passed by. He would raise his eyebrows suggestively. He would then look up with a wink and a nod each time he instructed the surgical technician to remove blood from the chest cavity by commanding her to "Suck." So, as soon as the doctor started to close, I hightailed it out of the operating room with the excuse I had a lunch meeting to attend. I wanted to avoid any additional uncomfortable exchanges or comments.

I would always wonder after that just what was being said and done without my knowledge when I was put under with anesthesia. This experience had certainly shaken my confidence in the professionalism of medical personnel. There was seemingly no sanctity in medicine, and no respect for the vulnerable. That saddened me.

Public Service for Maximum Profit

Another way in which pharmaceutical companies manipulate the market is through the support and financial backing of public service campaigns. Many nonprofit organizations that promote lowering cholesterol to reduce cardiovascular risk or inform you about the oppressive symptoms of social anxiety disorder (SAD) (not to be confused with another SAD, seasonal affective disorder) are doing so with funds donated by pharmaceutical manufacturers. Why? Because this type of advertising is highly effective with consumers who feel their best interests and improved health are the motivation behind these campaigns.

However, the truth is, although the nonprofit organization may indeed mean well, pharmaceutical companies are not charities. They are looking for a return on their investment. Overall, these programs are just well-disguised marketing campaigns designed to increase consumer awareness, thereby increasing drug sales for that disease.

The success of the latest marketing ploy of promoting diseases in lieu of drugs is self-evident. A perfect example of this emerged at the start of the psychopharmacological era, when Merck marketed the concept of depression along with amitriptyline "by buying and distributing 50,000 copies of Frank Ayd's book on recognizing and treating depression in general medical settings" (Healy, *The Antidepressant Era*, 181). In a similar manner, just as Eli Lilly was poised to launch Zyprexa, the nonprofit, consumer organization known as the National Alliance for the Mentally Ill (NAMI) began a massive campaign to educate the public about the prevalence of untreated mental illness. Booklets, pamphlets and other media were widely distributed to increase consumer awareness. What the public did not know was who was bankrolling this marketing effort and what they stood to gain financially. Reportedly, in a three-and-a-half-year period from 1996 to 1999, NAMI received $11.7 million in funding from drug companies. The largest donor during that time was Eli Lilly, who contributed $2.87 million. Eli Lilly's support also included an Eli Lilly executive who worked on loan at the NAMI headquarters, but whose salary was paid entirely by Eli Lilly (Levine 2).

Another such example is the 1999 Paxil Public Service Campaign. According to the Diagnostic and Statistical Manual of Mental Disorders—Fourth Edition (DSM IV), social anxiety disorder (SAD) is "an extremely rare condition" (Abramson 163). However, this public awareness campaign sponsored by Glaxo-SmithKline through three different nonprofit organizations—the American Psychiatric Association, Anxiety Disorder Association of America, and Freedom from Fear—helped get the word out about social anxiety and increase Paxil sales by twenty-five percent between 1999 and 2000. The initiative also won the distinction of Best P.R. Program of 1999 awarded by the New York chapter of the Public Relations Society (Abramson 163).

Direct-to-Consumer (DTC) Advertising

On any night of the week, count the number of pharmaceutical ads on television during prime time. Or, open your favorite magazine on any given subject. Count the ads. It is overload to say the least! "Ask your doctor about this…consult with your doctor about that." Nice, slick Madison Avenue ads feature happy, smiling faces of the medically challenged. What the pharmaceutical companies really mean is they want you to pressure your doctor into giving you their new drug. That way, they can influence his prescribing habits—yet once again—through you. A study conducted by the FDA in 2002 concluded that patients get prescriptions for drugs they requested more than fifty percent of the time. A *Prevention* magazine study printed in 1999 reported an even higher request rate of nearly eighty percent of the time (Abramson 156).

Now, a study that appeared in the *Journal of the American Medical Associ*ation on April 27, 2005, documents just how effective DTC advertising is in influencing patients to request particular antidepressants. The authors note that "antidepressant medications consistently rank among the top DTC advertising categories" (Kravitz). The study was designed as a randomized trial using standardized patients. The objective was to ascertain the effects of DTC-related requests on physicians' treatment decisions in patients diagnosed with depressive symptoms. The 152 doctors that participated were recruited from the San Francisco, California, and Rochelle, New York areas. The patients were middle-aged, white, and nonobese women. Most had professional acting experience. They were trained to present randomly to the doctors' offices between May 2003 and May 2004, portraying six different roles. The various scenarios included patients telling the doctor they had seen an ad on TV for Paxil and asking for the drug by name. Another might tell their doctor they had seen a show on depression and wondered if medication might be right for them. The researchers chose the SSRI Paxil because it is one of the higher-priced, more widely promoted antidepressant drugs.

As critics of DTC-advertising had already suspected, the authors found "antidepressant prescribing rates were highest for visits in which standardized patients made general requests for medication (76%), lowest for visits in which standardized patients made no requests for medication (31%), and intermediate for visits in which standardized patients the made brand-specific requests linked to DTC advertising (53%)." The results of this study "underscore the idea that patients have substantial influence on physicians and can be active agents in the production of quality," wrote the authors. "The results also suggest that DTC advertising may have competing effects on quality, potentially averting underuse, while also promoting overuse." Finally, they concluded, "The results of this trial sound a cautionary note for DTC advertising but also highlight opportunities for improving care of depression (and perhaps other chronic conditions) by using public media channels to expand patient involvement in care. [Here! Here!] Furthermore, physicians may require additional training to respond appropriately to patients' requests in clinically ambiguous circumstances" (Kravitz).

The excessive use of these DTC ads that rely on emotional appeals rather than medical evaluation and supply very little health information further undermines the patient-doctor relationship and the provider's clinical judgment about which drugs should or should not be used for the patient's medical benefit. It increases risk along with cost. However, the pharmaceutical companies argue these ads help improve public health by informing consumers and raising awareness. Proponents of the ads claim DTC advertising serves as an educational tool; even though, most of these ads vaguely describe the drug benefits in qualitative terms and then rarely support their claims with any clinical evidence (Kravitz).

Just remember, there are many older, less expensive drugs that have been around awhile. They also have much safer side effect profiles than the newer, highly promoted products. One of the reasons that Americans pay, on average, more than seventy percent more for our drugs than consumers in Canada and other countries is that DTC advertising of prescription drugs is not allowed in most foreign countries. Billions of dollars are spent annually on the advertising to create markets for branded prescription drugs. Which leads one to wonder: Exactly how medically innovative are these new products if they require such a massive effort to market? For example, Merck spent more than $160 million dollars in 2000 on DTC ads for Vioxx alone. In 2003, industry spending on DTC advertising totaled $3.2 billion (Kravitz). Those advertising expenses were passed on to you, the consumer. That would perhaps explain why expenditures for prescription drugs over the past several years have been increasing seven times faster than the rate of inflation (Abramson 245).

Also, contrary to what people may think, the FDA does not review DTC ads for accuracy and false claims before they are aired or published. When a manufacturer is found to be in violation by misrepresenting product benefits or risks, it has historically taken the FDA as long as one year to get the ads pulled or revised. A proverbial slap on the wrist is all that the company usually receives. When fines are levied, they rarely equal the positive financial impact the misleading ad has made for the company. Apparently, the long arm of the law does not reach as deeply as some of the pockets in this industry do.

The Smoke Screen of R & D Costs

If there is a mantra shared among all drug manufacturers, it is the catchall excuse of the high cost of research and development (R & D). As predictable as a beauty contestant's desire for world peace in any pageant interview, it is the automatic response each rep in the industry gives to exorbitant pricing complaints. In fact, they are almost smug about costs. "After all, you get what you pay for, right?" Of course, that statement would suggest to the doctor that the older products, now available generically, are in some way inferior to the newer, more costly products. "You do want cures to be found for cancer, AIDS, heart disease, and Alzheimer's, don't you? Well, who's going to pay for that?"

The truth is, one way or another, you are! However, it probably won't be through the outrageous prices you pay on prescription drugs. It will more than likely be through your tax dollars and the grants bestowed to the few tireless scientists and researchers who truly are in search of these cures as their mission in life. Moreover, the cures to our greatest medical fears probably won't come from a pharmaceutical company's laboratory either. Why? It does not benefit the pharmaceutical manufacturers to cure our diseases and restore our health and vitality. That's why!

Pharmaceutical companies are not the great humanitarian organizations we might want to believe they are. These executives don't rise to their morning coffee every day bursting with philanthropic desire to heal the world. They are businessmen who are accountable to stockholders and are basically motivated by bottom-line profits. Healthy profits! As my first regional sales manager pointedly told me in my final interview, "If it's altruism that motivates you, kid, join the Peace Corps. But, if it is money that motivates you, let me show you how you can retire a millionaire with this job!"

Drug manufacturers maximize their profits by treating our symptoms. The more long-term the illness is, the more profitable the treatment with drugs.

Just What the Doctor Ordered

Most of us think of drug dealers as the seedy characters that hang out in our schoolyards and back alleys trying to lure our children into drug addiction or as the rich Colombian warlord who runs a cocaine empire with machine guns and cash payoffs. The truth is that some of the most lethal drug dealers wear suits and ties, drive company fleet vehicles, and live in your very own neighborhoods. More importantly, they are addicting you and your children to the drugs they sell via your most trusted relationships—those with your doctors!

For the most part, pharmaceutical reps are attractive, personable, engaging sales professionals. The industry boasts of spending nearly $100,000 initially to hire, train, and indoctrinate a new rep. Basic sales training classes are much like boot camp and are designed to weed out the faint of heart or easily intimidated. (Working with the egos of doctors can wear on even the strongest self-esteem!) Trainers push new recruits to the breaking point, often giving them long hours of homework assignments into the night and weekends, videotaping sales presentations, and testing medical product knowledge. The environment is highly competitive as most reps desire to excel in front of their colleagues and educators. Not surprisingly, large numbers of these new hires cannot endure the stress and do not complete all tiers of their training. Only the most tenacious and ambitious succeed in having long-term careers in the industry.

Unfortunately, many reps come from other sales backgrounds that have little or nothing to do with either health care or medicine. Take me for example. Before joining the pharmaceutical industry in 1985, I had not so much as taken a chemistry or biology course. My undergraduate degree is a bachelor of arts in foreign language, Portuguese and Spanish. Although I consider myself intelligent and a fast learner, I was at first unequipped with the knowledge I needed to have even a basic understanding of the disease states and physiology or pharmacology involved in the drugs I was selling. That meant I was completely reliant on the product managers and marketing department for the accuracy of the information I gave doctors.

We were instructed to promote our products in a given manner and with a particular focus. This was called marketing direction. Individual thinking and style was definitely discouraged. Sales literature and visual aids were all geared toward the promotional message, and they were utilized in role-plays until the presentations flowed naturally. Reps were taught to handle and minimize the objections physicians might have. They were given the specific wording that would best represent the company's position. Often, these instructions came from the legal department who would review the sales documents for legal accuracy. If a visual aid initiated too many negative questions from physicians, the bar graph, product comparison, and so forth was reworked in a way that presented the information in a more favorable light. I had already learned the manipulative advantage of semantics in language, and I soon learned the semantics of research were called statistics.

Most doctors would deny the influence that sales reps have on their prescribing behavior. However, the fact of human nature is that we tend to support people that we like and feel are supportive of us. The pharmaceutical industry knows this all too well, and it provides the means for busy doctors to be accommodated in their practices by helpful, attentive sales professionals. These reps not only provide lunch, medical education, tools and devices, medical textbooks, calendars, scratch pads, and pens, but they also influence the doctors' personal lives. Reps make generous contributions to office parties, fund-raisers, and golf tournaments. They provide tickets to local sporting events and entertainment venues, and they coordinate social events such as boating, fishing, and hunting expeditions disguised as CME opportunities.

For example, if one of my doctors was too busy for me to gain regular access to his practice, I would invite the doctor and his wife or family to dine with me and a key opinion leader (KOL) in the community (a supporter of mine, of course). One time, I remember leasing a private room at a four-star Italian restaurant.

That afternoon, I sent a singing Italian waiter to the doctor's office with a bottle of champagne as a reminder and an invitation to him, his son (who was also an HVP with his own practice), and their wives to join my husband and me for dinner. I paid a local specialist, whom I knew to receive the majority of my HVP's referrals, $1,000 to have dinner with us and initiate a roundtable discussion about my product with the two family practitioners. The evening would more than pay for itself because both doctors increased their prescriptions more than twenty-five percent in the next three months. Prior to that, I had made very little impact on either lucrative practice. This practice of hiring KOLs to influence other doctors is quite common, and reps openly refer to these hired guns as prostitutes or drug whores because they are willing to sell their reputations to drug companies in this manner.

I have also known reps that joined a particular health club or church in order to gain casual access to a HVP who was difficult to access. One former colleague even babysat for a doctor's children in order to win his favor. I have sent doctors singing telegrams from various entertainer look-alikes, and I once had a belly dancer snuck into a hospital cardiac cath lab for a cardiologist's birthday. I was definitely a rep that was known as a goodie girl, and I never went anywhere empty-handed. I showered my giveaway items and promotional treasures on anyone and everyone in my path. For holidays and special events, I would make up goodie baskets around the theme of the occasion (for example, Easter, Halloween, or Christmas) and fill them with chocolates and gimmick items for office staff. On any given day or visit, there was always a trail of evidence from the latest marketing plan in my wake.

Why do some reps go to such great lengths to access and influence physicians? Pharmaceutical companies provide lucrative incentives for reps who reach sales quotas, and a rep stands to make several thousand dollars in one lump sum as a bonus in addition to his or her quarterly salary. Merchandise from catalogs and trip incentives are common as well. Over the years, I have won a Nikon 35mm camera, a Sony camcorder, a telescope, stereos, a set of luggage, a VCR, a Maytag washer and dryer, a daybed, company car upgrades, parasailing lessons, a weekend getaway package, and a trip to Hawaii with my spouse. I prided myself in my ingenuity, and I used creative, unique approaches to gain airtime with busy doctors and meet company sales goals. With my work ethic and enthusiasm, I advanced quickly in my career.

Legislative Attempts at Regulating Gift-Giving

At least fourteen states have introduced bills this year that would require pharmaceutical sales reps to file reports with their companies that detail the gifts they give to physicians. Of course, manufacturers are opposing the bills. PhRMA spokeswoman Wanda Moebius said the bills require manufacturers to disclose "trade secrets." She also claimed the laws are unnecessary because PhRMA already prohibits the practices lawmakers are attempting to curtail with its professional code of conduct (Robeznieks).

Most of the legislation restricts the reporting requirement to drug manufacturers, so medical societies have been reluctant to get involved because it will not affect the administrative responsibilities of doctors. According to the National Conference of State Legislatures, bills have been introduced in Connecticut, Illinois, Massachusetts, Nevada, New Hampshire, New York, Oregon, Rhode Island, and Washington. So far, only Maine and Vermont have succeeded in passing reporting laws. In five other states, the legislation has already been defeated (Robeznieks).

Learning That Ingenuity Sells!

My most successful, self-initiated sales campaign (and a perfect example of what I am discussing here) was in 1991 during the Gulf War. My husband had been deployed to Saudi Arabia, and everyone was talking about the war. It was difficult to conduct business under the circumstances. Nobody wanted to talk about drugs! So, I devised a "GI safety campaign" around Naprosyn, my new enteric-coated product, and utilized the war as my theme. I made all of my visits dressed in my husband's desert camouflage uniform and distributed miniature American flags and lapel pins everywhere I went. My lead-in to each sales presentation was the likening of a doctor's battle with disease to war and the necessity of ensuring GI safety in order to win that battle. Thus, the enteric-coated benefit (GI safety from ulceration) of Naprosyn provided the perfect bridge and play on words. My close to each presentation was an appeal for the doctor's support of my business while my husband supported our country abroad. My Naprosyn sales went through the roof after that! Less than one month after my husband returned home, I was promoted to an ob-gyn specialty rep's position and relocated to Austin.

The majority of drug companies know just what the doctor ordered, primarily because they subscribe to prescription data service companies that provide their sales force with detailed information on what doctors are prescribing in their practices. Pharmacies sell the doctors' prescription information, allowing companies to pinpoint who is supporting their product line and who is not. Reps frequently know more about a doctor's prescribing habits than he does himself! This data often verifies what marketers already know, and that is, when detail activity or call averages are increased in a doctor's office, the result is generally an increase in prescriptions for the products being promoted. The more memorable the presentation or information the doctor receives, the larger the assumed impact.

It would take many years and dozens of conscience-altering experiences before I really comprehended the scope of just how much my profession affected the medical industry and the contribution I had made to harming thousands of trusting people.

14

Related Current Events

"Intelligence is our first line of defense."

—Pres. George W. Bush

Recently, several investigative reporters have uncovered examples of questionable promotional strategies and incriminating documents distributed by pharmaceutical companies to their sales force. These documents instructed reps to dodge and/or minimize serious side effects or complications associated with their products. One such example appeared in the *Primetime Live* special on antidepressants ("Drug Company Investigation") that I referenced previously. ABC obtained marketing instructions issued to Paxil reps to minimize withdrawal side effects of the drug to doctors. Another appeared in a *60 Minutes* piece aired in November 2004. A paper trail uncovered by CBS revealed instructions for the intentional dissemination of misleading information in association with the Merck drug, Vioxx ("Prescription for Trouble").

With annual sales of more than $2.5 billion before being pulled from the market on September 30, 2004, Vioxx was one of the most successful new drugs ever launched. It was no small wonder considering the barrage of TV ads and unprecedented amount of direct-to-consumer advertising Merck employed (Appleby and Krantz).

Merck voluntarily pulled Vioxx after a new study showed the risk of heart attacks and strokes had doubled in the patients taking the drug. The document *60 Minutes* obtained was a training manual entitled "Dodge Ball Vioxx." It consisted of a twelve-page list of objections that could be posed by physicians. Among them was the objection, "I am concerned about the cardiovascular effects of Vioxx." A former Merck rep was quoted in the interview as saying, "We were supposed to tell the physician that Vioxx did not cause cardiovascular events, that instead, in the studies, Naproxen has aspirin-like characteristics which made Naproxen a heart-protecting type of drug where Vioxx did not have that heart-protecting side" ("Prescription for Trouble").

However, Naproxen has never been proven to have cardioprotective features like aspirin, and it has itself drawn negative attention in the same National Institutes of Health study that exposed the Cox-2 cardiovascular risks. At least two studies sponsored by Merck drew red flags early on to the cardiovascular and stroke event increases: the 1999 VIGOR (Vioxx Gastrointestinal Outcomes Research) study and the unpublished 1998 Study "090." (It is not uncommon for drug companies to claim their studies are "proprietary information" of economic value, thereby keeping the outcomes a secret.) Both studies showed an alarming (as much as sixfold) increase in cardiovascular events, including heart attack and stroke.

An estimated 20 million Americans took Vioxx in the five-and-a-half years it was on the market ("Prescription for Trouble"). Dr. David Graham, a lead investigator of the Cox-2 drugs, estimates Vioxx was responsible for an additional 88,000 to 140,000 deaths from cardiovascular ailments from 1999 to 2004 ("Merck Tried to Quash Vioxx Study").

The Cox-2 inhibitors remain in the news because, despite the numerous risks and marketing improprieties revealed surrounding Vioxx, it appears the FDA will allow them to stay on the market. This follows an advisory committee vote of 17 to 15 that agreed, for some people, the benefits of Vioxx outweighed its risks. That certainly should help limit Merck's liability price tag, which some analysts estimated to be $18 billion or more (Spake). The panel vote for Bextra was 17 to 13 with two abstentions. An overwhelming majority voted for the continued marketing of Celebrex at 32 to 1. According to the Center for Science in the Public Interest, ten of the panel experts who voted on these drugs had financial ties to the makers of Cox-2 inhibitors (Merck, Pfizer, Pharmacia, and Novartis) and had received honoraria, consulting fees, or research money from one or all of them. The majority of these experts voted in favor of the continued marketing of all the Cox-2s, including Bextra and Vioxx (Harris and Berenson).

The FDA was quick to refute critic's claims that panelists were "too cozy with drug makers" in a written rebuttal statement, claiming the agency had adhered to "strict ethics guidelines" in its screening of the advisory panel members for conflicts of interest. However, it went on to say that sometimes a "panelist's scientific expertise outweighed any potential financial interest" (Rubin).

It is apparent to me that our nation's health and safety have taken a backseat to the government's regulatory conflict of interest with the pharmaceutical industry. The problem has come full circle and threatens the health and welfare of everyone in this country. Absolutely, no one—man, woman, or child—is exempt!

The Complicity of Big Business in Government

The close affiliations between government and the pharmaceutical industry are legendary and the fodder of numerous scandals. Some of these relationships have had significant impact on legislative outcomes and government-funded research initiatives. Connections with Eli Lilly run deep in the current administration and date back to former President George Herbert Walker Bush, who was a member of the Eli Lilly board of directors at one time. Vice President Dan Quayle was another big player in Eli Lilly politics. Quayle is from Eli Lilly's home state of Indiana, and Eli Lilly was a major contributor to Quayle's senatorial campaigns (Breggin, *Toxic Psychiatry*, 151). When Quayle announced he would be running as the Republican vice-presidential candidate, the individual who made the announcement was Mitchell Daniels, Eli Lilly's vice president for corporate affairs. Daniels directed "government relations while advising the Bush-Quayle campaign on media strategy on nights and weekends" (Tracy 320).

Mitchell Daniels is also President George W. Bush's former director of management and budget. Sidney Taurel, a member of Bush's Homeland Security Advisory Council, is the current CEO of Eli Lilly. That might explain how legislation protecting Eli Lilly and other big pharmaceutical houses from litigation involving thimerosal ended up buried within the reams of paperwork comprising the Homeland Security Act. That's right: *New York Times* columnist, Bob Herbert reported this fact only days after its signing on a stowaway provision that defended makers of thimerosal, a preservative in vaccines that contains mercury and has been found to be a plausible contributor in the development of autism with children. Both Democrats and Republicans were so embarrassed by the disclosure that the provision was readily repealed (Levine).

Donald Rumsfeld, the secretary of defense in the Bush Administration, has enjoyed a lucrative career bouncing between government positions and the pharmaceutical industry. Before his current position in government, he was chairman of the board of Gilead Sciences, a biopharmaceutical company. He was also previously on the board of directors of Amylin Pharmaceuticals from 1991 to 1996 (News). Perhaps his most controversial affiliation was as chairman and CEO of G.D. Searle from 1977 to 1985, when he was hired to facilitate the FDA approval of aspartame (Equal, NutraSweet). Rumsfeld had reportedly vowed to his sales force he would "call in all of his markers" to get aspartame approved as a food additive. Rumsfeld was successful, of course, even though the FDA had opposed the approval of aspartame for sixteen years because of studies that showed it caused brain tumors and lesions in animals. Moreover, he received a $12 million bonus for his successful efforts with aspartame (Turner).

With the incoming Reagan administration was the appointment of a new FDA Commissioner, Dr. Arthur Hull. Commissioner Hull first approved aspartame, against the advice of FDA researchers, as a dry food additive. As his last act as commissioner before resigning his office in November 1983 to become senior medical advisor of Searle's public relations firm, he approved aspartame as an additive for soft drinks, in spite of the fact the National Soft Drink Association (NSDA) strenuously protested against it. The NSDA proclaimed aspartame to be "inherently, markedly and uniquely unstable" ("NSDA Protest"). The significance of that statement becomes relevant once you learn the pharmacology (and toxicology) of aspartame. It has a synergistic effect of transforming other substances such as ephedra, MSG, and pharmaceuticals into toxic compounds. Aspartame itself becomes a lethal poison (methanol) when broken down by the body.

Why does the pharmaceutical industry have such a stranglehold on American government? It is called noise level, and this industry knows the importance of noise level, especially in Washington DC. That's why they have more representatives than we do. That's right, the pharmaceutical industry employs more lobbyists to vocalize its position and protect its interests than we American citizens have representing us in the entire House of Reps and Senate combined. Of course, there are also hefty financial incentives provided to support politicians that pave the way for industry-supported legislation.

Did you know Republican Billy Tauzin, who led the House of Representatives committee that regulates drug makers, became the head of the Pharmaceutical Manufacturers Association (PhRMA), the most influential lobbying group for the pharmaceutical industry, in January 2005? Tauzin was deeply involved in the development of Medicare prescription drug legislation that showered billions of dollars on the pharmaceutical industry while doing nothing to halt increasing drug prices. Among the many issues Tauzin will be expected to lobby against is the cheaper import of drugs from Canada. The pharmaceutical industry is opposed to the legalization of imports from other countries. Tauzin voted against it in the House of Representatives last year. It is estimated Tauzin's salary will be $2 million dollars a year or more ("Tauzin Turns Top Drug Lobbyist").

Government Mental Health Screening Initiatives

Clearly, better mental health care is needed in this country. However, current initiatives by the President's New Freedoms Commission on Mental Health (NFC) to screen Americans for mental health issues and promote costly psychiatric drugs via treatment recommendations are grossly misguided. The commission suggested that the government start this initiative with our nation's 52 million schoolchildren. The NFC also supports a preferred drug program modeled after the Texas Medication Algorithm Project (TMAP) that was instituted when Bush was governor of Texas. The fact is, the main customers for these mandated drug treatment programs are the tax payers who fund state Medicaid budgets. TMAP was adopted in Texas in 1995. The state welfare system was in serious financial trouble by 1998. In 2002-2003, Texas lawmakers had to allocate an additional $1 billion for health and human services. A large portion of those funds were used to pay for prescription drugs (Pringle).

Aside from the exorbitant cost to state and federally-funded programs, I have already documented the abuse and overuse of psychiatric drugs on state-sponsored children in foster care in Texas. Dr. John Breeding, an Austin psychologist and Ritalin researcher, reported he has seen cases where some foster children were on as many as seventeen drugs. He agrees that drugs are being used as chemical restraints in Texas.

FDA Gets Mixed Reviews

The FDA has received a lot of criticism in the news lately about its handling of the Vioxx affair and over a recent survey that was conducted two years ago but just released in December 2004. The Public Employees for Environmental Responsibility obtained a copy of the survey through the Freedom of Information Act (FOIA) and published the study's findings, much to the dismay of the FDA.

The survey sampled approximately 400 FDA scientists about the evaluation and approval process of drugs and raises significant issues about drug safety and the ongoing monitoring of adverse events once drugs are on the market. As of two years ago, sixty-six percent of the participants surveyed said "they were not at all confident" or only "somewhat confident" the FDA adequately monitors the safety of prescription drugs once they are on the market ("Inside the FDA").

Unfortunately, unaware of what these regulators know, some Americans may still be overconfident in the FDA's ability to ensure the safety of prescription drugs. According to a survey conducted by the Kaiser Family Foundation in early February 2005, a large majority (eighty percent) remain confident of the safety of the drug supply. Furthermore, seventy-seven percent of those surveyed thought the FDA was doing a good job of ensuring drug safety. Although the survey revealed that consumer approval of the pharmaceutical industry overall was down, seventy-eight percent said that the use of prescription drugs makes a "big difference" in people's lives. Ninety-one percent felt pharmaceutical companies contribute significantly to society by the research and development of new drugs (Kaufman).

In his testimony to the Senate Finance Committee last November, Dr. David Graham raised concerns about several other prescription drugs he feels are dangerous to consumers and warned these drugs should either be restricted in their clinical use or removed from the market. They included the following: Meridia, the weight loss drug that has been linked to high blood pressure and stroke; Crestor, the lipid-lowering agent that has been known to induce renal failure in some patients; Accutane, the acne drug that has been linked to suicide, as well as other psychiatric symptoms (including psychosis) and birth defects; Serevent, the asthma drug that was shown in a long-term trial to cause death from asthma with ninety percent certainty; and Bextra, the Cox-2 inhibitor similar to Vioxx that has also been shown to increase the risk of heart attack and stroke ("FDA Denies Oversight Lapse").

Graham told Congress the FDA's problems with ensuring drug safety were "immense in scope" and left the American people "virtually defenseless" against the chance that dangerous drugs will reach consumers (Spake).

Recent Drug Recalls and Label Changes Issued

Obviously feeling the heat of the recent controversy, another Cox-2 inhibitor bit the dust on April 7, 2005. The FDA and European regulators requested that Pfizer remove Bextra from the market in the United States and European Union. The regulators cited "rare but serious skin conditions" as well as increased cardiovascular risk associated with Bextra as the reasons. They went further to say there was "lack of any demonstrated advantages for Bextra compared with other NSAIDs." (U.S. Food 2005c).

Pfizer was quick to "respectfully disagree with the FDA's position regarding the overall risk-benefit profile of Bextra" and vowed to do additional research on the heart problems affiliated with the Cox-2 class. Pfizer said it planned to have further discussions with the FDA and will try to bring the drug back (Cass). Well, of course it will! Pfizer sold $1.3 billion of Bextra in 2004. Celebrex, the last remaining Cox-2 on the market, is another Pfizer product that sold $3.3 billion last year ("Pfizer Takes Bextra Off Market"). FDA has also requested that Pfizer discontinue direct-to-consumer ads for Celebrex.

At the same time, the FDA is also recommending all drugs in the NSAID class carry a black box warning stating that "long-term use may cause cardiovascular side effects or gastrointestinal bleeding." This includes all prescription as well as over-the-counter NSAIDs, such as Advil, Aleve and Motrin (U.S. Food 2005c).

In late February, Tysabri, a new drug indicated for the treatment of multiple sclerosis (MS), was voluntarily withdrawn by its manufacturer after one patient died and another developed progressive multifocal leukoencephalopathy, a serious disease of the central nervous system. FDA approved Tysabri in an accelerated status after initial studies showed it reduced MS relapses by sixty-six percent compared to placebo. Biogen executives said about 5,000 people have received Tysabri since the drug's approval last November (Jewell).

The FDA has requested that Crestor's label be revamped to include a warning for Asian-Americans, patients with renal dysfunction, and those on cyclosporine that advises the starting dose be reduced to 5 milligrams daily. (Crestor is one of the newer statins that is frequently advertised direct-to-consumer.) A recent clinical trial discovered blood levels of Crestor in Asian-Americans were double those of Caucasians when administered at the same dose. This increases the risk of rhabdomyolisis, a serious muscle disorder that can lead to kidney failure. Rhabdomyolisis cases resulting in the death of fifty-three people were responsible for the removal of Baycol from the market in 2001. Baycol was a statin drug previously made by Bayer (U.S. Food 2001).

It is particularly troublesome that the FDA would allow a dangerous statin drug to remain on the market, especially when elevated cholesterol is considered a risk factor (not a disease) and these drugs are only used as preventative treatments intended to improve health and increase longevity. The jury is still out among physicians as to the validity of excessively lowering cholesterol and if decreasing their patient's low density lipoprotein (LDL) levels below 100 is necessary, as stipulated by the latest clinical guidelines last revised in 2001.

In 2002, the *Journal of the American Medical Association* published a study that found four out of five participants in the formulation of clinical practice guidelines had financial ties to pharmaceutical companies. The authors of the clinical guidelines on cholesterol were no exception. Moreover, the majority of these decision makers had active financial relationships with the makers of the very drugs affected by these guidelines.

Cholesterol is vital to many of the body's functions and is the most common organic molecule in the brain. More importantly, it is also an essential building block of some of our most important hormones, such as stress hormones, blood sugar-regulating hormones, and sex hormones. When one looks at all the data, another little known phenomenon is revealed about this whole business of lowering cholesterol: The risk of death from all causes other than coronary heart disease increases significantly with lower total cholesterol levels for both men and women after the age of fifty (Abramson 133-134).

15

An Ounce of Prevention or a Pound of Cure: It's Your Choice!

"The doctor of the future will give no medicine, but will interest his patients in the care of the human frame, in diet, and in the cause and prevention of disease."

—Thomas A. Edison

There are no quick fixes to maintaining a healthy body and brain. Health is a lifelong pursuit and commitment. Eating a balanced, nutritious diet, getting regular aerobic exercise, drinking enough water, getting adequate amounts of quality sleep, and taking nutritional supplements for your individual health needs is a great place to start. Unfortunately, with the stress of our modern culture and lifestyles, these preventative health measures alone are not enough. According to my chiropractor, Dr. David Armstrong, this is why:

> Your brain continually produces messages in the form of electrical impulses that travel throughout the nervous system to the cells in the body. The nerves, located between the vertebrae (spinal bones), are the nerves that carry messages from your brain to all the body's organs and tissues. This is a two-way communication process from the brain to the body cells and from the body back to the brain cells. Every single body function is completely under the control of your nervous system. Anything that interrupts this flow of communication can be detrimental to your health, mental and physical.

When a vertebra shifts out of alignment, it can put pressure on the spinal nerves interrupting the flow of energy within the body. This is known as subluxation. Subluxation interferes with your body's ability to heal and lowers immune response. Any imbalance in one area of the spine causes other areas of the spine to work harder in order to compensate for the area out of balance. This can lead to disease.

Continual pressure on the spine from prolonged standing or sitting; the impact of walking, exercise, or trauma; gravity; and daily tension from emotional and physical stress contributes to vertebral subluxation. In addition, chemical toxicity from drugs, food, and the environment can cause reflexive stress to the spine. Therefore, maintaining a healthy spine, which is the housing of the central nervous system, through regular chiropractic care keeps the body's life energy flowing properly. This, in turn, facilitates healing and strengthens the immune system and your body's ability to neutralize allergens, viruses, and bacterial pathogens.

Mood Disorder and Sleep Deprivation: Get Your Beauty Sleep!

I am one of the luckier "walking wounded" diagnosed with a mood disorder. Fortunately, I have only experienced two subsequent hypomanic episodes in the twelve years following my antidepressant-induced manic psychosis. Once again, both were attributable to prescription drug use. One episode was moderately severe (and, coincidentally, marked my fortieth birthday and a visit from my sister, Michelle). The other was a fairly mild response to benzodiazepines that I had been given in anesthesia and post-surgically to sleep. I didn't even realize I was hypomanic until the episode had passed, and I was left to deal with some very embarrassing behavior.

Sleep deprivation is as much a precursor to manic episodes as it is a result of them. Because I know that and because I have an ever lingering fear of becoming manic, I'm very protective of my sleep. I am very picky, in particular, about my sleeping environment, for example, mattress, room temperature, darkness, soundproofing, and so forth. Sleep is a sacred ritual for me. I wind down every evening with a warm aromatherapy bath or shower (this assists the body temperature to drop more quickly and helps you fall asleep), listen to soothing music, take herbal supplements to help me relax about an hour before bedtime (Gaia Herbs makes an excellent formulation called Sound Sleep), and conclude my day with meditation and prayer. If I am really caught up in the monkey chatter going on in my head, I make a "to do" list of all the day's unfinished business in order to release the burden of remembering it until the next day. Then, I write down a list of the day's frustrations or challenges and the people who have hurt or angered me in some way. One by one, I consciously release them all with love. Finally, I make a list of the things I am grateful for and do an *Om* meditation to quiet and clear my mind and expand that feeling of gratitude. By the time I'm finished, I am generally centered enough to relax and achieve a deep and restful night's sleep.

I have found these natural rituals and therapies to be much more beneficial to my health than taking prescription hypnotic sedatives that are known to be highly addicting. One cautionary note: Melatonin is another popular natural sleep remedy, but melatonin has been known to induce mania in some susceptible individuals.

If you like to walk or exercise and, hopefully, you do, try to do so as early as possible. Exercise starts my engine, so to speak, and it generally is not a good idea for me to do it too late in the day. It can delay my ability to fall asleep. If I fail to have any other time except the evening to incorporate exercise, I skip the aerobic exercise. Instead, I do a few gentle yoga poses designed to relax the body and mind and stretch the spine and musculature.

What the Real SAD Public Awareness Campaign Should Be About

Unfortunately, because no particular industry is able to capitalize on the profits of improved health and longevity, there is very little incentive to inform the public about the impact the Standard American Diet has on our health and well-being. The acronym for the American diet is very appropriate, SAD. There has been an explosion of type 2 diabetes diagnosed in our nation over the past decade. Currently, more than 16 million Americans suffer from diabetes, and another 24 million are said to have preclinical diabetes. More tragically, the average age of onset with type 2, which used to be called adult-onset diabetes, has drastically decreased. Where once type 1 (or juvenile diabetes) was the only type of diabetes seen in children, children are now being diagnosed with type 2 every day in the United States (Abramson 228-230).

This is due in no small part to the nutritionally depleted American diet that consists largely of processed foods, refined carbohydrates, and cholesterol-laden fats in toxic quantities. The lack of whole fresh foods, particularly fruits and vegetables, and the consumption of massive amounts of additives and sugar has exhausted our adrenals, weakened our immune systems, and set us up metabolically for chronic fatigue, anxiety, insomnia, diabetes, obesity, allergies, depression, attention deficit disorder, cardiovascular disease, and many other diseases.

The brain is a finely tuned instrument that cannot function without the proper fuel and environment for neuronal transmission. Many micronutrients are needed for the brain and the central nervous system to work optimally. Many of those nutrients must be derived from foods, because the body cannot manufacture them itself. Most of us do not consume the seeds, berries, fish, and other marine life that supply these essential nutrients for our brain. Therefore, not only do we consume too many of the wrong things, but we do not eat enough of the right things either! These micronutrients are the building blocks for health and mental well-being. Without these building blocks, our bodies and minds are unable to adapt to the stressors we encounter in our environment. The result may be aberrant behavior or physical illness that can be directly linked to metabolic and subsequent brain malfunction caused by poor nutrition.

Poor dietary habits run in cultures and, therefore, in families. Children who live on cereal, Pop-Tarts, potato chips, bologna sandwiches, macaroni and cheese, soda pop, and candy bars and families who get their meals carried in or at the fast-food drive-up window are the norm in America, not the exception. We are creating our own nutritional nightmare. We are one of the wealthiest, developed nations on the planet, and we are malnourished. According to the World Health Organization, we have more health problems and worse health outcomes than many underdeveloped, impoverished nations. Now that is sad!

Omega-3 Fatty Acids: Phenomenal Brain Food

I would be remiss not to mention the groundbreaking discovery made by the Harvard researcher, Dr. Andrew Stoll, in the utilization of Omega-3 essential fatty acids in the treatment of a variety of psychiatric disorders, including depression, bipolar disorder, attention deficit/hyperactivity disorder, and even violence. In his book, *The Omega-3 Connection*, Dr. Stoll convincingly takes us through the history and evolution of man and his diet and shows us how altering our once abundant, natural consumption of fish, crustaceans, and other sea life has halted our evolution as a species. We are deficient in the single nutrient most responsible for a healthy brain and body, Omega-3 fatty acids. Omega-3 fatty acids fall into the category of polyunsaturated fats. These fats are very good for us when they're not highly processed or overheated. Omega-3 fatty acids are found in cold-water fish, soybeans, organic eggs, almonds, sunflower seed, pumpkin seed, flaxseed, and their oils.

Plenty of clinical data substantiates the benefit of Omega-3 fatty acids in the treatment and prevention of Crohn's disease, arthritis, cardiovascular disease, and diabetes. Dr. Stoll's research on the treatment of bipolar disorder with Omega-3 fatty acids was published in 1999 in the *Archives of General Psychiatry*. His research concluded that Omega-3 fatty acids have remarkable therapeutic value in the treatment of bipolar illness, even the most chronic, resistant cases (Stoll 23).

A very recent scientific study conducted by Oxford University's department of physiology appeared in the *American Journal of Pediatrics* in May 2005. The study found that forty percent of children made dramatic improvements in reading and spelling when taking Omega-3 supplements. The data also showed a significant improvement in concentration and behavior. Symptoms often associated with attention deficit/hyperactivity disorder were reduced significantly, usually as much as would be anticipated with a prescription drug such as Ritalin. Although no specific data about other health improvements was published in the study, it did mention that parents had reported improvements with other health problems such as eczema and asthma as well (Lawrence).

Results of this research validate the suspicions of parents and teachers everywhere. Children's diets are inadequate for their basic development needs. The average American junk food diet and our approach to the treatment of children's behavior disorders with addictive stimulants is the ultimate closet abuse of our nation's children.

Knowledge Is Power: Learn to Speak Medical-ese

If you have a chronic illness (or are the primary caretaker of a loved one with a chronic illness) that requires you to have frequent interaction with doctors and other medical personnel, learn their language. Improving communication can minimize your risk. Don't be intimidated by your provider's medical vocabulary. Learn it! Enter your diagnosis into any Internet search engine, and read to your heart's content. If you don't have a computer, access one at your local school or library. You can also buy books on the subject to gain additional insight and exposure to medical terminology.

Armed with the knowledge gained from a little research, you will feel more confident and comfortable asking questions. You will also be better capable of comprehending your doctor's findings and treatment plan. Once you learn to communicate with your health care professionals, you can partner in your healing and health maintenance process rather than blindly submit to the mandates of others. Don't be afraid to speak out, ask questions, or, if necessary, challenge authority! Nobody knows your body better than you. Ultimately, you will pay the health consequences for errors in diagnosis and treatment, as well as the hefty financial bill.

I know many wonderful doctors whom I admire and respect, but they are just men and women like you and me. They have specialized skills and education and speak a language specific to their trade, but so do lawyers, plumbers, mechanics, accountants, and computer programmers, among others. I can't stress enough that MD does not stand for "medical deity." Doctors are people, not Gods! They have human motivations and weaknesses. They are fallible. They make mistakes.

And as I have just shown you, they are often deliberately misinformed by enterprising pharmaceutical companies and their representatives.

Find a Spiritually-based Support Network

If your network of immediate family and friends does not provide the emotional support you need, involve yourself in a spiritual network, community, or church. Relationships we choose with healthy, like-minded individuals are much more rewarding than those dysfunctional ones we retain out of a sense of obligation or guilt. It is important to surround yourself with compassionate, caring people that empower rather than impede your life and growth process. Rod and I have found our church and clergy to be a wonderful source of strength, advice, support, education, and spiritual resources in times of marital difficulties and personal challenge.

Herbal Medicinal Alternatives

My transition into sales and management in the natural foods industry these past five years has been another eye-opening experience. It has given me an education on various supplements, herbs, and vitamins. Probably the most important thing I have learned is how closely medicinal herbs mimic pharmaceutical activity in the human body, especially when those herbs are standardized isolates from a total plant compound.

For example, when I was still selling statins (cholesterol-lowering drugs), the pharmaceutical industry was lobbying the FDA to have a natural red yeast rice product, Cholestin, pulled from the market. The reason given was that Cholestin was so effective in lowering cholesterol that it performed like a pharmaceutical in the body. So, the industry's argument was that Cholestin should have been classified as a drug and subjected to all the clinical testing and rigors required by such. The industry's lobby was successful, and the FDA agreed. Cholestin was pulled from the market, effectively removing yet another competitor and natural alternative to the pricey, toxic pharmaceuticals currently used to lower cholesterol.

Consumers often take for granted, even though herbs may be a more natural approach to healing, there are also risks of adverse reactions and drug interactions, just like there are with pharmaceuticals. It is important to inform your health care provider about all of the remedies (prescriptions, over-the-counter drugs, herbs, vitamin supplements, and so forth) you are taking in order to avoid unnecessary reactions.

There are many excellent herbal alternatives to prescription pharmaceuticals. Unfortunately, a few bad apples have given the natural health industry a black eye. As with anything else, buyer beware! Do your homework before purchasing herbal products. Find out who the reputable companies are. The supplement industry is self-regulated, and quality varies significantly from manufacturer to manufacturer.

My last employer, Gaia Herbs, makes liquid extracts and vegetarian phytocaps utilizing a full spectrum standardization process of each plant compound. This allows the natural buffers of the plant to remain in balance with other standardized components. Gaia Herbs is a pharmaceutical-grade, GMP-certified facility that manufactures exceptionally high quality medicinal herbs for retail trade and naturopathic physicians. It is one of the few companies in the United States that still produce kava kava, my current herbal aid in the ongoing battle against anxiety.

When given justice, the scope and depth of the information about alternative treatments for depression and other psychiatric illnesses, including herbs, is a book in and of itself. So, because of the urgent nature of this information, I will not delay publication of this book to include it. I will, however, write a sequel that addresses beneficial herbs and other natural therapies for mental wellness.

CONCLUSION

So, WHAT EXACTLY IS THE TRUTH?

"Truth has no special time of its own. Its hour is now—always."

—Albert Schweitzer

I don't know if people are becoming more educated about bipolar illness and, therefore, more people are getting diagnosed because of increased awareness, but there has definitely been an increase in recent years in the number of people who either know someone who is bipolar or have themselves been diagnosed with the disorder. When I was growing up, hardly anyone I talked to had ever heard of it before. I would go to great lengths to try to explain the family defect.

Now, bipolar disorder appears to be the latest diagnostic vogue in psychiatry. Headlines scream of increases in the mentally ill. An article in the *Austin American Statesman* cited a seventy-nine percent increase in mental health diagnoses in twenty Austin-area hospitals and health clinics from 2003 to 2004. In Texas, this was due in part to the shuffling of the mentally ill from inpatient to outpatient settings and the budget cuts ordered by Gov. Perry in community mental health centers (Ball). However, this mental health dilemma is not unique to Texas.

Mental illness diagnoses are on the rise nationally, as evidenced by the massive increase in psychiatric drugs sold in the United States. Is it really mental illness that is on the rise? Could there be a correlation with the increase of mental symptoms and the increased use of antidepressants and other psychoactive drugs? Remember, any psychiatric drug can induce the symptoms it is designed to treat in many people.

Is the American medical community creating new chronically ill mental patients with excessive prescribing of psychoactive drugs? Does the American diet have a causal relationship along with these drugs in the explosion of diabetes in our population? Is the pharmaceutical industry fueling this psychiatric diagnostic frenzy, thereby perpetuating the problem with public awareness campaigns and direct-to-consumer advertising that sends us clamoring into the doctor's office requesting the latest magic pill to fix our mental angst, our aching back, our

142

chronic fatigue, our sleeplessness, and our social anxiety? Are doctors receiving fair, balanced education on these drugs and their potential side effects?

I can't help but play a fantasy scene in my head of some ambitious product manager mocking a novice, Eli Lilly rep who might have posed the naive question, "Since initial clinical trials were only four to six weeks in duration, doesn't that mean there could be increased risk associated with the long-term use of Prozac?" by pompously chuckling and responding, "Well, of course it does. But, luckily for those people, we have an excellent atypical antipsychotic in the pipeline called Zyprexa!"

Just as a closing reminder and final food for thought on this subject, Zyprexa has been shown to cause diabetes, right? Well, luckily for its stockholders, Eli Lilly's second-largest income is derived from its diabetes care products that grossed more than $2.61 billion in 2004 (Swiatek).

My Personal Truth

"Healing is of God in the end…Revelation may occasionally reveal the end to you, but to reach it the means are needed."

—A Course in Miracles

In accepting personal responsibility for my own health, I have renewed hope in the future. Biopsychiatry had bashed those hopes into oblivion at one time, convincing me I was genetically damaged goods and would never be normal again without drugs. Had I completely succumbed to that diagnosis, I'm certain my outcome would have been different. It may take a redefinition of normal to say I beat the odds, but I have learned that psychiatry is highly subjective anyway. What may seem like eccentric behavior to some is defined as pathology by others. My goal is the same as Hippocrates, "do no harm" to anyone (including myself) and help as many people as I can.

I have found acceptance in being unique, at least with myself and in a community of like-minded individuals. With the love and support of my husband and son, now sixteen years old, I feel extremely blessed and humbly grateful for my life. I have redefined success as well. I feel more successful today than I ever have, even though I no longer have a lucrative, high-profile sales job, simply because I no longer feel the need to impress anyone. I honor my spirit, listen to my heart, and try to always follow that gut feeling. I am very content to just "be" in the moment now. I take time to stop and smell the roses.

After several of my acquaintances had read this book, they questioned how I had turned out so normal. I have to smile because I know some of them thought I may have included a few too many personal anecdotes about my life and strayed a little from the thesis. (Someone told me all authors tend to take that liberty.) However, all of the events I have written about, however seemingly irrelevant to my subject matter, had significance to me because of that very question: How did I turn out so normal, and why was I spared some of the more serious ramifications from my poor choices? These events further illustrated the answer to another question: What relevance did some of these things have in my development and final outcome?

I have prayed about my life considerably and, in particular, about these questions. This is what I have received: I am not normal. I am special. All human beings are. I have special gifts, special talents, special sensitivities, special challenges, and a special calling. These things are all blessings. None should be misinterpreted as punishment or a curse that has been inflicted upon me. All are the result of my own choices. If I had not "lived" these things, I may never have found the capacity for compassion and forgiveness that has ultimately expanded my awareness and freed my wounded spirit.

My experience was all part of my learning and growth process. The challenges made me stronger and a more creative problem solver. The education gave me a vast array of knowledge about a variety of health subjects and therapies that help me manage the damage done to my brain by drugs. The multitude of opportunities I have had gave me the tools to succeed in my life's mission. Even the silly beauty pageants I hated so much had a divine purpose. They taught me how to interview, stage presence and poise in front of an audience, and how to swim with the sharks (compete with cutthroat competitors). They also gave me confidence, as well as public speaking skills.

As for my foreign exchange experience in Brazil, that exposed me to a loving, supportive family environment at the age of sixteen. It was an experience that gave me a multitude of blessings, starting with a functional example to model my own family by. It also gave me the exposure to college that later motivated me to attend and better my opportunities through higher education. Finally, it gave me the security and self-confidence to literally embark on the journey of exploring the world. I have been to eleven other countries and nearly every state in the United States. (Incidentally, we also received a wonderful Brazilian student in our home from 1999 to 2000. This was another spin-off of this remarkable experience for me.)

The original intent of this book was not to write about my family or expose the skeletons in my closet. It was my plan to write an exposé about antidepressants and, of course, include my personal perspective and experience in the pharmaceutical industry. However, after Meg died and I was so acutely reminded of the continuing familial dysfunction that had scarred all of our lives, I began waking to an urgent dictation in my head. It was a storyline connecting all of my life events, just as God had done in our meeting in the wee morning hour ten years ago. Although I felt resistant to inflicting more emotional pain on myself and the ones I love, I knew this was the book I was supposed to write. I had to write the story that was in my heart, the story that had led me down this path and to this realization. It was the truth that would honor Megan's life and death, and it was the truth that would set me free.

So, this has been my personal account of an odyssey in education and self-discovery, my journey of faith and forgiveness. It is my life story—warts and all! Many of these events nearly broke my heart, but none of them has broken my spirit. I have asked God for forgiveness for my anger, weakness, and fear. But mostly, I have sought forgiveness for the love I have withheld from others because of my pain. After all, the only way love can possibly hurt you is if you don't give it away. I have forgiven each and every one who has ever transgressed against me. It is my prayer that anyone I have hurt intentionally or unintentionally will do the same for me. It's true that forgiveness is for the *forgiver*, not the *forgiven*.

I apologize to those loved ones who may not be pleased about having their dirty laundry aired in public. But your stories are an integral part of my story. They could not be omitted and still paint the picture of family dysfunction as it truly exists. There was no malicious intent behind any of these disclosures. You are the only family I have, and I love you all unconditionally.

If my story gives one family or even one person the courage to stand up and make personal choices to heal rather than medicate their psychological wounds, then it was worth it. If one desperate soul finds solace or inspiration in our shared experience, then it was worth it. If one child's life or brain is spared destruction, then it was worth it! My hope is that other families may learn from our mistakes and this autopsy of the soul will serve to educate future healers. The truth is, as human beings, we are all doing the best we can with what we have to work with under our individual circumstances. At least, that is my truth!

What Can We Do To Change Things?

What is to be gleaned from all of this information? Hopefully, I have made my case for the need to accept personal responsibility for one's health and mental wellness. It should also be obvious that our country needs to develop a real, unadulterated, evidence-based medicine approval and regulatory system. We must make our disgust about the financial conflicts of interest that threaten our families and their health known to our legislators and resolve only to support those politicians committed to affect change in our crippled, deadly, health care system.

To assist in that effort, I have established a Web site at www.gwenolsen.com that links to a site with the current names and addresses of every state's representatives, as well as form letters you can print, sign, and forward to your local senator or congressman. This will make it easy and convenient to vocalize your concerns about these issues. As new information becomes available, I will update the Web site to reflect it. Please do your part, however large or small you deem appropriate. If nothing else, give someone this information after you read it. Inform one more soul, and I will be satisfied.

I pray this information has clearly illustrated that, when we attempt to reduce our moods or behaviors to simple brain chemistry, not only do we ignore the scientific evidence, we ignore the spiritual evidence that would suggest otherwise. We know so little about the origin and treatment of mental disorders, and history has taught us in hindsight that some theories and treatments in medicine can be dead wrong! (Just look at the hormone replacement debacle with women.)

At a minimum, it should be apparent that our current health care system is in desperate need of revamping and, particularly, our approaches to the treatment of mood disorders and other mental illness with toxic, harmful chemicals should be critically reevaluated, if not discouraged. Finally, the facts, rather than marketing fiction, about each of these treatments should be thoroughly disclosed to the patients and their caretakers. Not only is it a matter of informed consent, it is a matter of public safety. I seriously doubt, when given the full scope of the risk being taken, that many patients who are currently on antidepressants for minor physical ailments (such as, chronic pain, weight loss, and so forth) would continue to take them or many loving, concerned parents would opt to go this route for their troubled children or adolescents.

There Is Hope!

Everything in life is as it should be, and it has always been so. In *A Course in Miracles*, it says, "Nothing real can be threatened. Nothing unreal exists. Herein lies the peace of God" (Foundation for Inner Peace, Preface *x*). We may not always understand or agree with the direction of the course of events in life. However, when we accept that everything happens for a reason, we find ourselves more intuitively tuned in to which path to follow when we come to a fork in the road. If we take the path less traveled, we are often pleasantly surprised. If we force ourselves to overcome fear and resistance, it generally results in a huge payoff. Yes, sometimes, even financially!

Surrender is our greatest strength in this life experience. To just "let go and let God" can be very difficult at first. But when we use it as a powerful transformative tool and an affirmation of love and trust in the goodness of the universe and God's special plan for each of us, we can make a conscious commitment every day to learn subsequent life lessons in mild and gentle ways through a daily invocation and surrender to God's will. It becomes easier and easier with every miraculous outcome we experience.

When we allow our internal navigational system to be placed on autopilot, it flawlessly leads us from one circumstance to the next, one relationship to the next that is required for our continued growth and learning. We always have the free will to alter God's plan, but when we do, the course is typically a little choppier than necessary. You know what they say, "If you want to hear God laugh, tell him your plan!"

When we assume personal responsibility for our actions and the outcome of events in our lives, rather than blaming others, we empower ourselves to change those things we find unsuitable to our needs. We then realize we are in charge of what we experience. As such, we achieve psychological healing. In victim consciousness, we remain encumbered by a feeling of powerlessness. We blame our consequences on circumstances or influences without, rather than looking within to find the real cause and solution to our problems. Drugging our emotions into submission only further compounds our feelings of hopelessness. Why? Because if we never make a conscious decision to change, nothing around us ever changes!

> *Life is a gift.*
> *Open it with exuberance!*
> *Tear at its bright bows and colored paper*
> *with enthusiasm and expectation.*
>
> *Know that what lies inside*
> *may not always be what you asked for,*
> *but it is a gift none-the-less.*
> *Therefore, be humbly grateful...*
> *Be inspired to give back.*

Every day is a new chance to celebrate
the wonder of life
and the mystery of love.

You cannot reinvent perfection
and in God's eyes you are perfect
just the way you are.

Love yourself as you learn to love others.

Honor your spirit
and the individual qualities
that make you uniquely you.

And remember…
Every life you touch is a life you can serve.
By being the difference
you can change your world!

—Gwen Olsen

Now, I turn it all over to you, dear God. Thy will be done on earth as it is in heaven. Amen.

GLOSSARY

Adolescence: the stage in human growth from the onset of puberty to the attainment of full physical development

Adrenaline (epinephrine): a hormone that prepares the body for danger or stress

Adverse Event: a pharmacologic term that refers to a negative reaction caused by a drug

Agitation: an extreme emotional disturbance in which someone is highly perturbed

Akathisia: a neurological state of inner restlessness that is extremely uncomfortable and involves involuntary motor hyperactivity, for example, pacing, fidgeting, foot tapping, and so forth

Anticholinergic: a drug that inhibits the action of a parasympathetic nerve

Anti-inflammatory: a pharmacologic agent used to relieve inflammation and pain

Anxiolytic (benzodiazepine): a pharmacologic anti-anxiety agent that produces sedation by reducing central nervous system activity

Antidepressant: a pharmacologic agent used specifically to treat depression by increasing neurotransmitter levels in the brain and interfering with their reuptake

Antidote: an agent that counteracts the effects of an ingested poison, either by inactivating it or by opposing its action following absorption

Antagonist: a substance that reduces or blocks the action of another substance or of some physiological process

Antipsychotic (neuroleptic): a pharmacologic agent used to treat psychotic symptoms such as hallucinations and delusions

Autoerotic Asphyxiation: a form of sexual self-arousal and self-gratification from suffocation

Bipolar Disorder (Manic Depression): a mental disorder usually involving mania and/or hypomania and alternating periods of depression. There are three major types of bipolar illness: Bipolar I, Bipolar II, and Cyclothymia.

Bipolar I: the classic syndrome of mood swings in which manic symptoms begin gradually and become increasingly worse. Psychotic symptoms may accompany the manic episodes. A mild, brief period of depression usually follows a manic episode. Some people experience symptoms of mania and depression simultaneously. This is referred to as a "mixed" episode. Mood irritability is a predominant component of the illness.

Bipolar II: expressed primarily as depression, which can last for several months at a time. Symptoms of mania that do occur may be brief and very mild.

Blood-Brain Barrier: the protective lining shielding the brain from chemical substances

Borderline Personality Disorder: a pervasive pattern of instability of interpersonal relationships, self-image, affects, and marked impulsivity beginning by early adulthood

Buccalfacial Tics: involuntary neuromuscular movements involving the tongue, cheek, mouth, and face

Central Nervous System (CNS): the body system that consists of the brain and spinal cord and communicates messages throughout the body to the brain and vice versa

Cortisol: an important stress hormone that prepares the body to respond to danger or stressful situations

Cyclothymia: a mood disorder that is characterized by milder mood swings that tend to be more brief in duration than Bipolar I symptoms

Delusion: a false belief that is held in spite of invalidating evidence

Depression: emotional dejection; morbid sadness accompanied by loss of interest in surroundings and a lack of energy; generally includes sleep disturbance

Dopamine: a monoamine neurotransmitter that is essential to normal nerve activity. It is specifically associated with some forms of psychosis and movement disorders.

Dysphoria: an emotional state characterized by depression, restlessness, and malaise; usually accompanied by poor self-esteem.

Encopresis: the unintentional passage of feces

Endocrine System: a bodily system consisting of several ductless glands that secrete hormones into the blood. It includes the thyroid gland, the adrenal glands, the sex glands, and the pituitary and pineal glands. This system communicates with the body's organs and tissues and controls their functioning.

Endogenous: means it is biologically based; anything found with the body

Endorphins: a group of peptides normally found in the brain and other parts of the body; capable of producing effects similar to those of opiates

Exogenous: means it is externally based; anything originating from the environment

Generic: term used when referring to the nonproprietary name of a drug

Genome: a complete set of chromosomes (with their genes) from one parent; the total genetic endowment

Gestational Diabetes: an insulin-resistant disorder that occurs during pregnancy

Glucose: a form of sugar present in most plant and animal tissue that is the major energy source of the body

Grandiose (grandiosity): a term in psychiatry denoting feelings of great importance; having delusions of grandeur

Hallucination: the perception of objects or events that do not exist

Homeostasis: a state of physiologic equilibrium in the body (for example, temperature, blood pressure, chemical content, and so forth)

Hypnotic (sedative): a pharmacologic agent used primarily to induce sleep. Hypnotics produce sedation by reducing central nervous system activity.

Hypomania (hypomanic): a moderate form of manic activity, usually marked by slightly abnormal elation and overactivity

Kindling: a learned aberration of brain chemistry that begins with a stressor that triggers an episode. This kindling process increases vulnerability to further stress and can lead to further episodes.

Lability: means instability or the condition of being changeable

Limbic System: an important group of brain structures comprising the cortex and related nuclei near the brain stem, which are thought to regulate emotion, behavior, memory, and certain aspects of movement, such as facial expression

Lobotomy: the surgical severance of nerve fibers connecting the frontal lobes to the thalamus for the relief of some mental disorders

Mania (manic): an emotional disorder characterized by a state of excitement, hyperactivity, and profuse and rapidly changing ideas

Mood Disorder: a condition in which the primary feature of illness is mood disturbance; may also affect thinking and behavior

Narcissism: a psychiatric term that refers to the excessive admiration or love of self

Narcotic: a pharmacologic agent that is intended for the relief of pain that also tends to produce insensibility, stupor, and sleep. With prolonged use, it may become addictive.

Neuroleptic (antipsychotic): a pharmacologic agent used particularly in the treatment of psychosis and schizophrenia

Neurons: the cells that are the basic structural units of the nervous system. They transmit one-way electrochemical messages to and from the brain. Unlike most cells, they cannot divide and cannot be replaced.

Neurotransmitter: a chemical messenger that relays information between adjacent nerve cells in the body

Norepinephrine: a neurotransmitter related to epinephrine that is found in both the peripheral and central nervous systems. This is the neurotransmitter that arouses the fight-or-flight response when the body experiences stress.

Paranoia: a rare, slowly progressive mental disorder characterized by convincing and logical delusions of persecution and grandeur without any other signs of personality deterioration

Placebo: an inert substance containing no medication but prescribed as medicine, given especially to satisfy a patient. It is also used in controlled studies to determine the efficacy of drugs.

Prefrontal Cortex: the front one-third of the brain that affects attention span, impulse control, judgment, as well as organization and problem-solving skills

Psychiatrist: an MD who specializes in psychiatry and primarily biopsychiatry, which involves treatment with drugs

Psychologist: a mental health professional that holds an advanced degree in psychology. These professionals cannot prescribe medication and generally provide patients with talk and/or other forms of psychotherapy.

Psychosis: a severe mental illness of organic and/or emotional origin, marked by loss of contact with reality and frequently by regressive behavior, delusions, or hallucinations

Rapid Cycling: a bipolar state in which manic or hypomanic and depressive symptoms alternate during a single day or from day to day

Receptor: a term in pharmacology that refers to a constituent in a cell that combines with a specific drug, resulting in a change of the cell's function

Reuptake: the reabsorption by a neuron of a neurotransmitter following the transmission of a nerve impulse across a synapse

Schizoaffective Disorder: a combination of schizophrenia and mood disorder

Schizophrenia: a category of severe emotional disorders marked by disturbances of thinking including misinterpretation of reality and sometimes delusions and hallucinations. There are associated changes in mood and behavior, particularly withdrawal from people.

Serotonin: a neurotransmitter found in the central nervous system and peripheral ganglia. It is implicated in several mental disorders, including depression.

Tardive Dyskinesia: a drug-induced disorder that causes involuntary repetitive movements known as tics, such as muscle spasms, writhing or twisting, and odd facial expressions and mouth or tongue movement

Tics: involuntary, brief, and recurrent twitching of a group of muscles, most commonly involving the face, neck, and shoulders

Thyroxin: a hormone produced in the thyroid gland and is responsible for maintaining a normal metabolic rate in all the cells of the body

Tricyclics: a category of antidepressant drugs that possess three rings in their molecular structure, such as imipramine, amitriptyline and doxepin hydrochloride

BIBLIOGRAPHY

Abramson, John. *Overdosed America: The Broken Promise of American Medicine.* New York: HarperCollins, 2004.

Angell, Marcia. *The Truth about the Drug Companies: How They Deceive Us and What to Do about It.* New York: Random House, 2004.

Avorn, Jerry. *Powerful Medicines: The Benefits, Risks, and Costs of Prescription Drugs.* New York: Alfred A. Knopf, 2004.

Bradshaw, John. *Family Secrets: The Path to Self-Acceptance and Reunion.* New York: Bantam Books, 1995.

Breggin, Peter R. *Toxic Psychiatry.* New York: St. Martin's Press, 1991.

———. *Talking Back to Prozac.* New York: St. Martin's Press, 1994.

Breggin, Peter R. and David Cohen. *Your Drug May Be Your Problem.* Cambridge: Da Capo Press, 1999.

Cohen, Jay S. *Over Dose: The Case Against the Drug Companies.* New York: Jeremy P. Tarcher, 2001.

Drummond, Edward. *The Complete Guide to Psychiatric Drugs: Straight Talk for Best Results.* Canada: Wiley, 2000.

Foundation for Inner Peace. *A Course in Miracles.* California: Foundation for Inner Peace, 1977.

Fried, Stephen. *Bitter Pills: Inside the Hazardous World of Legal Drugs.* New York: Bantam Books, 1998.

Glenmullen, Joseph. *Prozac Backlash: Overcoming the Dangers of Prozac, Zoloft, Paxil, and Other Antidepressants with Safe, Effective Alternatives.* New York: Touchstone, 2000.

Goozner, Merrill. *The $800 Million Pill: The Truth behind the Cost of New Drugs*. Berkeley: University of California Press, 2004.

Healy, David. *The Antidepressant Era*. London: Harvard University Press, 1997.

————. *Let Them Eat Prozac: The Unhealthy Relationship between the Pharmaceutical Industry and Depression*. New York and London: New York University Press, 2004.

Kassirer, Jerome P. *On the Take: How Medicine's Complicity with Big Business Can Endanger Your Health*. New York: Oxford University Press, 2005.

Kuhn, Cynthia, Scott Swarzwelder, and Wilkie Wilson. *Buzzed*. New York and London: W. W. Norton & Company, 1998.

Reed Stitt, Barbara. *Food & Behavior*. Manitowoc: Natural Press, 1997.

Stoll, Andrew L. *The Omega-3 Connection*. New York: Simon & Schuster, 2001.

Strand, Ray D. *Death by Prescription: The Shocking Truth behind an Overmedicated Nation*. Nashville: Thomas Nelson Publishers, 2003.

Tracy, Ann Blake. *Prozac: Panacea or Pandora?* West Jordan, Utah: Cassia, 2001.

————. "Our Serotonin Aftermath," unnumbered materials in *Prozac: Panacea or Pandora?* West Jordan, Utah: Cassia, 2001.

Valenstein, Elliot S. *Blaming the Brain: The Truth about Drugs and Mental Health*. New York: The Free Press, 1988.

Whitaker, Robert. *Mad in America*. Cambridge: Perseus Publishing, 2002.

Whybrow, Peter C. *A Mood Apart*. New York: HarperCollins, 1997.

REFERENCES

Desk Reference to the Diagnostic Criteria from DSM-IV-TR. Washington, DC: American Psychiatric Association, 2000.

Melloni's Illustrated Medical Dictionary. 2nd ed. Baltimore: Williams & Wilkins, 1985.

Physicians Desk Reference. Montvale, New Jersey: Medical Economics Company. 2000.

Taber's Cyclopedic Medical Dictionary. 19th ed. Philadelphia: F. A. Davis, 2001.

The Holy Bible, New International Version. Grand Rapids: Zondervan Bible Publishers, 1973.

ARTICLES AND BROADCASTS

Appleby, Julie and Mark Krantz. 2004. Merck Estimates $2.5B Impact from Pulling Vioxx Plug. *USA Today,* October 1.

Ball, Andrea. 2005. Hospitals Seeing More Mentally Ill. *Austin American Statesman,* January 23.

Boyles, Salynn. 2005. Suicide Rate Down on Prozac. *CBS News WebMD,* February 2.

Cass, Connie. 2005. Pfizer Takes Painkiller Bextra Off Market, FDA Wants Warnings on Others. *Associated Press,* April 7.

Cassidy, Frederick, Eileen Ahearn and J. Carroll.1999. Elevated Frequency of Diabetes Mellitus in Hospitalized Manic-Depressive Patients. *American Journal of Psychiatry* September; 156: 1417–1420.

DeGrandpre, Richard. 2002. The Lilly Suicides. *AlterNet,* Aug 22, 2002. http://www.alternet.org/envirohealth/13893/(accessed February 20, 2005).

DeNoon, Daniel. 2004. Child Antidepressant Use Skyrockets: Use Growing Fastest in Preschool Kids. *WebMD,* April 2, 2004. http://my.webmd.com/content/Article/85/98399.htm (accessed June 20, 2005).

"Dr. Glenmullen's Q & A: Antidepressant Side Effects." ABC News Online. December 9, 2004. http://abcnews.go.com/Primetime/print?id=333966 (accessed December 15, 2004).

"Drug Company Investigation." ABC News *Primetime Live.* December 9, 2004. Broadcast.

"Drugs on the Brain." *WORLD Magazine.* October 12, 2000.

"FDA Denies Oversight Lapse." CBS News. November 19, 2004. Broadcast.

"Forced Drugging." *AAPS News* 58.5 (2002).

"Friend: School Shooter on Prozac." CBS News. March 26, 2005. Broadcast.

Gardner, Amanda. 2005. "Suspension of Adderall XR Sales Not Likely in U.S." *HealthDay News,* February 10.

Gardner, Fred. 2004. Eli Lilly's Bitch: The NIMH. *CounterPunch,* September 11/12.

Harris, Gardiner and Alex Berenson. 2005. 10 Voters on Panel Backing Pain Pills Had Industry Ties. *The New York Times.* February 25.

Huffington, Arianna. 1997. Peppermint Prozac. *U.S. News & World Report,* August 18.

IMS Health. 2005a. IMS Reports 2004 Global Pharmaceutical Sales Grew 7 Percent to $550 Billion. March 9 March 2005. <http://www.imshealth.com/ims/portal/front/articleC/0,277,6599_3665_71496463,00.html (accessed June 20, 2005).

———. 2005b. Looking to China and cancer as cost containment slows growth. March 30. http://open.imshealth.com/webshop2/IMSinclude/i_article_20050330.asp (accessed June 20, 2005).

"IMS Reports 9 Percent Constant Dollar Growth in '03 Global Pharma Sales." *ACRP Wire* April 2004: Vol. 2, Issue 4.

"Inside The FDA." CBS News. December 16, 2004. Broadcast.

Jewell, Mark. 2005. "Biogen, Elan Voluntarily Withdraw MS Drug." ABC News. February 28. Broadcast.

Kaufman, Marc. 2005. Drugs Get Good Ratings, But Drugmakers Less So. *Washington Post,* February 26, A03.

Ko, Marnie. 2003. The Downside of Drugs. *Undercover Medicine.* February. http://www.undercover-medicine.com/s5/s2/article74.shtml (accessed June 9, 2005).

Kotulak, Ronald. 2002. Experts Concerned over Extended Use of Anti-panic Drug. *Chicago Tribune,* October 21.

Kravitz, Richard L., et al. "Influence of Patients' Requests for Direct-to-Consumer." *Journal of the American Medical Association* 2005.293: 1995–2002.

Lawrence, Felicity. 2005. Children's Diet Link to Disorders. *The Guardian*, May 2.

Levine, Bruce. 2004. Eli Lilly, Zyprexa, & the Bush Family: The Diseasing of Our Malaise. *Z Magazine Online*. http://zmagsite.zmag.org/May2004/levine0504.html (accessed February 20, 2005).

"Merck Tried to Quash Vioxx Study." CBS News. January 25, 2005. Broadcast.

Nielsen, Susan. 2001. "The Doctor Made Me Do It." *The Oregonian*, July 1.

"NSDA Protest Summary." Congressional Record, Senate.7 May 1985: S5507-S5511.

"Pfizer Takes Bextra Off Market." *WCCO News*. April 7, 2005. Broadcast.

"Prescription for Murder." CBS News, *48 Hours*. April 16, 2005. Broadcast.

"Prescription for Trouble." CBS News, *60 Minutes*. November 14, 2004. Broadcast.

Pringle, Evelyn. 2005. "Bush Cheney 'Mental Health' For Kids: Take Drugs." Independent Media TV. May 28.

"Risks of Anti-Psychotic Drugs Eyed." CBS News. January 27, 2004. Broadcast.

RM News. 2005. Rumsfeld Lobbied FDA Approval of Toxic Aspartame. *Conspiracy Planet*. May 30. http://www.conspiracyplanet.com/channel.cfm?channelid=55 &contentid=107 (accessed May 30, 2005).

Robeznieks, Andis. "More States Consider Laws For Reporting Industry Gifts." *AMNews*. May 9, 2005.

Rubin, Rita. 2005. "The COX-2 Dilemma: Risking Heart Problems to Ease Pain." *USA Today*. March 3.

Spake, Amanda. 2004. "A Sick Agency in Need of a Cure?" *U.S. News & World Report*. December 13.

Springer, John. 2005. "In Attempts to Pin Killings on Zoloft, Some Unwelcome Statistics for Boy's Defense." Court TV. February 10. Broadcast.

Starfield, Barbara. 200. "Is U.S. Health Really the Best in the World?" *Journal of the American Medical Association,* 284 (2000): 483–485.

Swiatek, Jeff. 2005. Tax on Overseas Profit Fuels Loss for Eli Lilly. *Indianapolis Star,* January 27.

"Tauzin Turns Top Drug Lobbyist." CBS News. December 16, 2004. Broadcast.

Turner, James S. 2002. The Aspartame/NutraSweet Fiasco. Environment, Technology and Society Forum. August 25.

U.S. Food and Drug Administration (FDA). 2001. "Bayer Voluntarily Withdraws Baycol." August 9. http://www.fda.gov/bbs/topics/ANSWERS/2001/ANS01095.html (accessed April 23, 2005)

U.S. Food and Drug Administration (FDA). 2005a. "Alliant Pharmaceuticals Expands Its Voluntary Nationwide Recall of Methylin® CT, 2.5mg, 5mg, and 10mg Tablets" January 14. http://www.fda.gov/oc/po/firmrecalls/alliant02_05.html (accessed April 23, 2005).

U.S. Food and Drug Administration (FDA). 2005b. "FDA Public Health Advisory on Crestor." March 2. http://www.fda.gov/cder/drug/advisory/crestor_3_2005.htm (accessed June 16, 2005).

U.S. Food and Drug Administration (FDA).2005c. "COX-2 Selective (includes Bextra, Celebrex, and Vioxx) and Non-Selective Non-Steroidal Anti-Inflammatory Drugs (NSAIDs)" April 7. http://www.fda.gov/cder/drug/Infopage/COX2/default.htm (accessed April 23, 2005).

U.S. Food and Drug Administration (FDA). 2005d. "Deaths with Antipsychotics in Elderly Patients with Behavioral Disturbances" April 11 http://www.fda.gov/cder/drug/advisory/antipsychotics.htm (accessed April 23, 2005).

Wilde Mathews, Anna. 2004. Congress Will Discuss Drug Trial Issues. *Wall Street Journal,* September 8.

978-0-595-35763-5
0-595-35763-6

To Jo —

Blessings,
Dan Olsen

Printed in the United States
128482LV00002B/10/A

9 780595 357635